The Cleft Care Framework in India

Panchali Batra • Badri Thiruvenkatachari
Deborah Sybil
Editors

The Cleft Care Framework in India

A CCIS Report

Springer

Editors
Panchali Batra
Department of Orthodontics
Jamia Millia Islamia
New Delhi, Delhi, India

Badri Thiruvenkatachari
University of Manchester
Manchester, UK

Deborah Sybil
Dept of Oral and maxillofacial surgery
Jamia Millia Islamia
New Delhi, Delhi, India

ISBN 978-981-99-8970-6 ISBN 978-981-99-8968-3 (eBook)
https://doi.org/10.1007/978-981-99-8968-3

This Springer imprint is published by the registered company Springer Nature Singapore Pte Ltd.
The registered company address is: 152 Beach Road, #21-01/04 Gateway East, Singapore 189721, Singapore

Foreword

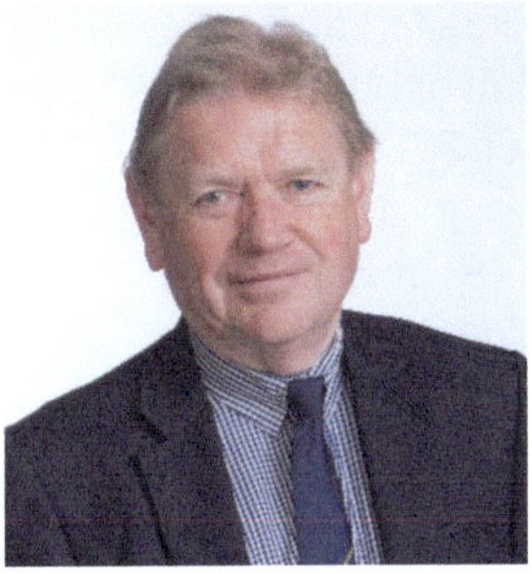

Children born with cleft lip and palate face a lifetime of difficulties with wide-ranging issues. Although this is the most common craniofacial anomaly in humans, the condition is not regarded as life-threatening and neither is the priority for treatment considered as essential in all healthcare systems. This has led to some children failing to have their cleft lips or palates closed early in life and as a result, these children have to cope, often in isolation, with difficulties in speech, hearing, oral function, facial appearance, and deeply traumatic psychological and psychosocial functioning. There are also impacts on the mother at birth and the rest of the family in providing a supportive environment for those children born with a cleft who then receive inadequate treatment.

The anomaly is a global issue with one child born with a cleft somewhere in the world every 3 minutes. The cause of the anomaly is unknown, but it is thought that genetic and environmental factors are involved. Several large groups work on these areas to try and establish the cause of clefting as well as develop potential strategies for prevention. Although these groups require extensive funding to conduct this research, the impact of their findings will not be realized for some time. There are growing pressures for both finance and staffing in healthcare systems, and cleft lip and palate care will only receive priority where a case for the importance of treating the condition is made. This requires healthcare workers and researchers who understand the condition and the importance of treatment to make a case to providers and the government to establish treatment centers. Typically, the service to treat these children is fragmented and dispersed with the consequence that the condition does not have all the necessary specialists available. The research that is needed to establish these priorities seems of low importance, yet if the condition is treated within a well-organized health care system that understands the existing literature on the care of these children, there are great savings for the providers and an enormous benefit to the child born with a cleft. Although the research needed to demonstrate the benefits of healthcare process and outcomes for cleft children born with cleft is poorly funded and difficult to do, Professor Panchali Batra has achieved this. The immediate impact of her findings will be significant if healthcare funders are willing to take notice.

A similar approach in the United Kingdom has achieved improvements in outcomes by up to 50%; system re-organization will achieve far more for this condition than any amount of money spent on genetic and environmental research. Professor Panchali Batra is to be congratulated for her remarkable research skills and courage in undertaking this work, which has the potential to make a significant impact on the lives of children born with a cleft.

Jonathan Sandy
FMedSci, PhD, FDS, Morth, (RCS England)
Emeritus Professor in Orthodontics
University of Bristol
Bristol, UK

Foreword

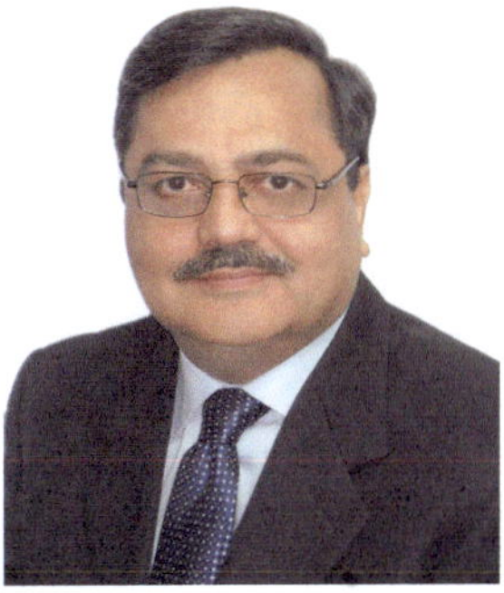

I am honored to write this foreword for a unique compilation on cleft care in India. I have known Panchali Batra for over a decade, and I have seen her grow as an excellent clinician, devoted teacher, and meticulous researcher.

Cleft lip and palate care is a topic that is very close to my heart. I am closely associated with promoting interdisciplinary cleft care through various forums and the Indian Society for Cleft Lip, Palate and Craniofacial Anomalies. I have travelled worldwide to learn and share cleft care logistics and science challenges. Cleft care in India needs to be reformed and implemented using a country- and context-specific strategy. I have faced challenges in interdisciplinary cleft care and require authentic information on the quality of treatment and treatment outcomes. To address this, India Cleft, a multicenter task force project funded by the Indian Council of Medical Research, laid the foundation for baseline data. Our efforts continued by initiating an advanced full-time fellowship in cleft orthodontics and enhancing a dedicated cleft care center at the Center for Dental Education and Research, All India Institute of Medical Sciences, New Delhi.

This exceptional and unique monograph evaluates the standard of cleft care in India. The monograph is based on real-life experiences from 19 cleft care centers located in various regions of India. The authors of this monograph have successfully highlighted the challenges faced while attempting to evaluate the standard of cleft care. Each center has a unique journey to share, be it supported by charitable non-governmental organizations or private hospitals. The monograph is divided into seven sections, with sections 1 and 7 being the most useful for readers. These sections provide an overview of the global burden of cleft, introduce the Cleft Care India study, and share observations from the young team of investigators.

This project was funded by the Ministry of Education under the SPARC scheme. Dr. Panchali Batra led the Indian investigation, and Dr. Badri T. served as the overseas investigator from the University of Manchester.

The gathered data sheds light on the cleft care status through well-formulated and comprehensive data assessing the patient through photographs, radiographs, surgical details, oral health, speech, voice recordings, intelligibility in context scale (ICS), and audiology evaluation forms. The cultural, social, and ethnic diversity much reflected in the distribution of cleft in different regions of India, the nutrition affecting and modifying the epigenetic influences and further literacy, education resources, the economy availability of experts influencing the age of surgery type of surgery, and other treatments provided to cleft children.

I congratulate the authors for this excellent, thoughtful, and timely compilation of data leading to comprehensive information that adds value to earlier work on the India cleft project, a task force project funded by ICMR that concluded in 2020. This compilation is a landmark work that sets a roadmap for the future of cleft care in India and low- and middle-income countries.

O. P. Kharbanda

MDS (Lucknow), M MEd (Dundee),
M Orth RCS (Edinburgh), FDS RCS
(Edinburgh), FDS RCS (England),
FAMS, British Commonwealth Fellow:
Cleft Orthodontics Manchester, Professor
of Orthodontics, Faculty of Dental Sciences,
Pro Vice-Chancellor-Health Sciences, Ramaiah
University of Applied Sciences, President-Ramaiah
Memorial Hospital
Bengaluru,India

Professor Emeritus and Council member,
National Academy of Medical Sciences,
Past President Indian Society for Cleft
Lip Palate, Craniofacial Anomalies,
Formerly : Prof and Head Orthodontics
and Dentofacial Deformities, Chief Centre
for Dental Education and Research,
All India Institute of Medical Sciences
New Delhi,India

Preface

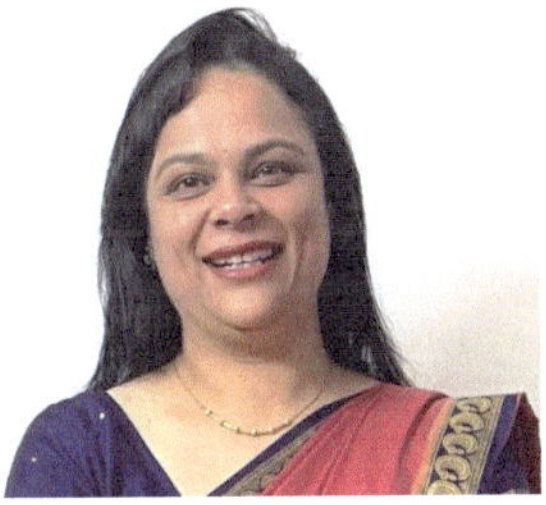

Caring for children afflicted with cleft lip and palate has been of utmost importance to me. This dream took its wings when a project under the Scheme for Promotion of Academic and Research Collaboration (SPARC) was sanctioned by the Ministry of Human Resource Development (now Ministry of Education), Government of India, to Jamia Millia Islamia. This was also the time when I first interacted with Dr. Badri through a common friend, Dr. Mohit affiliated to the University of Sheffield. Dr. Badri, an avid researcher and a thorough gentleman, was associated as Honorary Senior Lecturer in Orthodontics at the University of Manchester, UK. Manchester also happens to be a renowned institution revered for its notable and immense contributions to the realm of cleft research on a global scale.

This monograph serves as the outcome of the Cleft Care India Study, on which I have been working with my dear friend Dr. Deborah Sybil, oral and maxillofacial surgeon, since 2018. The idea of compiling the journeys and struggles of these centers came to us when Deborah and I were sitting beside each other on a plane journey to visit a few lead cleft centers in our country. This project allowed me to interact and collaborate with over 15 centers across India with the help of Dr. Puneet Batra who was then the president of Indian Society of Cleft Lip Palate and Craniofacial Anomalies. Professor Jonathan Sandy from University of Bristol, who was the lead of cleft care in the UK and the force behind the revolutionary centralization of cleft care services, extended his great support and shared resources beneficial for this project.

This monograph documents the developmental journey of the 19 state-of-the-art cleft care centers in India. The objective was to provide readers with a comprehensive overview of the challenges and progress accomplished by these organizations in establishing exemplary centers for the treatment of cleft lip and palate. In addition to their surgical accomplishments, these hospitals provide a wide range of in-house services aimed at promoting the overall well-being of their patients. A few of these institutions also contribute to the advancement of education by granting fellowships and actively engaging in research and innovations.

With varied funding sources, these healthcare centers ensure the provision of optimal and high-quality healthcare services to patients suffering from cleft and craniofacial deformities. Along with their noteworthy accomplishments, these centers encounter various challenges, such as the need for augmented human resources that are specifically trained in cleft care, including speech therapists, trained personnel for record-keeping, and paramedical staff. The absence of defined protocols and the lack of patient surveillance in the context of cleft care remain the areas that require improvement.

The journeys covered in this monograph possess the capacity to provide direction to those endeavoring to construct analogous infrastructure on a global scale. This book could help in addressing the lacunae in the current standard of cleft care which could be helpful to the Ministry of Health/Rashtriya Bal Swasthya Karyakram (RBSK) to formulate robust and comprehensive strategies for cleft care and surveillance in India.

B.D.S., M.D.S., M OrthRCS (Edinburgh, UK), FDSRCS (England),
Professor, Orthodontics and Dentofacial Orthopaedics,
Jamia Millia Islamia, New Delhi, India

Panchali Batra

Contents

Part I
Overview

Chapter 1
Global Burden of Cleft Lip and Palate

Deborah Sybil, Sakshi Katyal, Panchali Batra, Imran Khan, and Disha Garg

1.1 Introduction

Global Burden of Diseases refers to a "comprehensive demographic and epidemiological framework to estimate health gaps for an extensive set of disease and injury causes, and for major risk factors, using all available mortality and health data and methods to ensure internal consistency and comparability of estimates"[1]. GBD is an analytical tool that helps in identifying countries achieving success in meeting oral health goals, and thus identifies strategies to reduce the burden of oral health conditions. The burden of disease is different from the prevalence of disease and is calculated by years of life lost through premature death (YLLs) and years lived with a disability (YLDs). To capture the impact of both premature death and disability in a single measure, an internationally standardized measure is used—Disability Adjusted Life Year (DALY). DALY is a measure of the gap in healthy years of life lived by a population as compared with a normative standard [1]. For oral health conditions, DALYs reflect the YLDs only. YLDs are calculated by multiplying the frequency (prevalence), severity (disability weight), and duration of the condition [2].

According to the Global Burden of Disease Study 2019, the leading cause of burden globally in the age group younger than 10 years were infections related to lower respiratory infections, diarrheal diseases, malaria, meningitis, whooping cough, and congenital syphilis. Among 10–24 years, road injuries, self-harm, and

D. Sybil (✉) · I. Khan
Department of Oral Surgery, Faculty of Dentistry, Jamia Millia Islamia, New Delhi, India

S. Katyal · P. Batra
Department of Orthodontics, Faculty of Dentistry, Jamia Millia Islamia, New Delhi, India
e-mail: pbatra@jmi.ac.in

D. Garg
Faculty of Dentistry, Jamia Millia Islamia, New Delhi, India

P. Batra et al. (eds.), *The Cleft Care Framework in India*,
https://doi.org/10.1007/978-981-99-8968-3_1

interpersonal violence were the leading causes of burden. Ischemic heart disease and stroke were the top-ranked causes of DALYs in both the 50–74 years and 75 years and older age groups [3]. In India, the leading causes were ischemic heart disease, chronic obstructive pulmonary disease, diarrheal diseases, lower respiratory infections, and cerebrovascular disease [4].

1.2 Global Burden of Oral Diseases

According to WHO, 3.5 billion people globally, suffer from one or the other form of oral disease which means that the global burden of oral diseases is more than the combined global burden of the next five most prevalent non-communicable diseases [5]. Untreated Dental caries in permanent dentition contributed to 2.3 billion of this burden followed by severe periodontitis, untreated caries in deciduous teeth, and total tooth loss [6]. This data may not be a true representation of India since our country lacks state-level data for oral health diseases [7, 8].

Oral diseases add to a huge economic burden of approximately 710 billion US$ incurred at direct or indirect expenditures. Edentulism holds the highest global burden of about US $167 billion followed by severe periodontal disease which costs about US $82 billion.

1.3 Global Burden of Cleft Lip and Palate

Congenital malformations especially, undifferentiated orofacial clefts (estimated 4.6 million cases globally), noma and traumatic dental injury have a significant impact on the health and well-being of populations. Orofacial clefts are one of the most common congenital anomalies, but this disease burden is disproportionately distributed worldwide. This burden falls maximum on the countries with the smallest surgical workforce or with the lowest socio-demographic index [9].

The global incidence rate of CLP is approximately one in 600–800 live births (1·42 per 1000), and isolated cleft palate occurs 1 in 2000 live births. Among all the clefts, 15% are isolated cleft lip, 45% cleft lip and palate, and 40% are cleft palate alone [10], with unilateral clefts four times more common than bilateral and 70% being on the left side. Both the frequency and severity of clefting are higher in boys as compared to girls. The majority of the cleft cases (50%) are present as a part of syndromes (around 300 reported syndromes) such as Van der Woude syndrome, Pierre Robin syndrome, Treacher Collins syndrome, etc. and may be associated with other developmental abnormalities [11]. 40% of the cases show a familial history of clefts, a single cleft parent can lead to a 3.2% chance of having a child with cleft lip and palate and a 6.8% chance of having a child with isolated cleft palate. If one parent and one sibling are affected, then there is a 15.8% chance of cleft lip and palate and a 14.9% chance of cleft palate in the next child [12].

It is noteworthy that 4·62 million people are living with unrepaired or inadequately repaired cleft [13]. The prevalence of orofacial cleft was estimated to be 10.8 million, with a disease burden of 652,084 DALYs, with 94.1% of the disease burden in low- and middle-income countries [14]. Asians have the highest incidence of 0.82–4.04 per 1000 live births, followed by Caucasians, of about 0.9–2.69 per 1000 live births and the lowest incidence rate among Africans, of about 0.18 – 1.67 per 1000 live births According to a 2020 report by Institute for Health Metrics and Evaluation, around 600,000 children younger than 5 years of age had clefts, and among these, 200,000 were found to be underweight. Thus making them 2.15 times more likely at risk for growth failure compared to the general children under 5 years of age [13].

Cleft lip and palate have significant physical, psychological, social, and financial consequences for affected individuals. These families also experience social stigma, discrimination, and reduced opportunities for education and employment. Access to specialized healthcare services, including surgical interventions and multidisciplinary care, is often a challenge, especially in low-income groups. Apart from dental therapies, patients may undergo up to 20 surgeries through adolescence during cleft rehabilitation.

The unique anatomy of the lip and palate in these patients impacts the muscle coordination needed for swallowing due to the decreased ability to create suction during breastfeeding and bottle feeding, thus, increasing the possibility of food inhalation and aspiration, and also the time required for feeding. Dysfunctioning of the palate muscles results in the retardation of some consonant sounds and abnormal nasal resonance thus leading to speech difficulties and also making them prone to chronic ear infections.

Atypical dental development, malocclusion, presence of natal and neonatal teeth, microdontia, taurodontism, ectopic eruptions, delayed tooth maturation, and enamel hypoplasia are common dental findings in OFC patients.

1.4 Burden of Cleft Care in India

In India, a total of 0.033% of the Indian population suffers from OFC, which accounts for around 423,519 Indians having clefts, among which 226882 are males, and 196637 are females. Around 27,000–33,000 children with cleft are born each year. It is important to note that around 72,637 patients of OFC have an unmet need, which is 18.76% of the total Indian cleft population with OFC. The DALYs lost are around 2.05 for 100,000 males, 2.66 for females and 2.34 for both sexes [15]. The unmet needs are majorly limited to the lack of access to surgical care in India.

The impact of OFC is not only felt by the patients but also by their families. Burden of care and Medical poverty trap are the two terms to highlight the impact on families in India. The burden of care is much more than the DALYs, and it includes the loss of time and compromise in quality of life undergoing multiple interventions. In India, 60% of the population resides in rural areas, among these many patients are daily wagers. Each visit to the hospital means loss of his earnings plus out-of-pocket expenses on travel and treatment which can destroy the financial stability of the family.

Many non-government agencies have strengthened the surgical need, but comprehensive care and surveillance will take a long to establish in India.

References

1. Lopez AD, Mathers CD, Ezzati M, et al., editors. Global burden of disease and risk factors. Washington, DC, The International Bank for Reconstruction and Development/The World Bank; 2006.
2. GBD 2017 Oral Disorders Collaborators, Bernabe E, Marcenes W, et al. Global, regional, and national levels and trends in burden of oral conditions from 1990 to 2017: a systematic analysis for the Global Burden of Disease 2017 Study.
3. GBD 2019 Diseases and Injuries Collaborators (2020). Global burden of 369 diseases and injuries in 204 countries and territories, 1990-2019: a systematic analysis for the Global Burden of Disease Study 2019. Lancet (London, England).
4. India State-Level Disease Burden Initiative Collaborators (2017). Nations within a nation: variations in epidemiological transition across the states of India, 1990–2016 in the Global Burden of Disease Study. Lancet (London, England)
5. Nityanand Jain, Upasna Dutt, Igor Radenkov, Shivani Jain. WHO's global oral health status report 2022: actions, discussion and implementation. 20 January 2023
6. Dye BA. The global burden of oral disease: research and public health significance. J Dent Res. 2017;96(4):361–3.
7. Miglani S. Burden of dental caries in India: current scenario and future strategies. Int J Clin Pediatr Dent. 2020;13(2):155–9.
8. Batra P, Saini P, Yadav V. Oral health concerns in India. J Oral Biol Craniofac Res. 2020;10(2):171–4.
9. Massenburg BB, Hopper RA, Crowe CS, Morrison SD, Alonso N, Calis M, Donkor P, Kreshanti P, Yuan J. Global burden of orofacial clefts and the world surgical workforce. Plastic and reconstructive surgery. 2021;148(4):568e–80e.
10. Gaurishankar S. Textbook of orthodontics. 1st ed. Paras Medical Publication; 2011.
11. Allan E, Windson J, Stone C. Cleft lip and palate: etiology, epidemiology, prevention and intervention strategies. AnatPhysiol. 2014;4:1–6.
12. Banerjee M, Dhakar A. Epidemiology-clinical profile of cleft lip and palate among children in India and its surgical consideration. CIBTech JSurg. 2013;2:45–51.
13. Christensen K, Mitchell LE. Familial recurrence-pattern analysis of nonsyndromic isolated cleft palate—a Danish Registry study. Am J Hum Genet. 1996;58(1):182–90. PMID: 8554055; PMCID: PMC1914943
14. Massenburg BB, Hopper RA, Crowe CS, et al. Global burden of orofacial clefts and the world surgical workforce. Plast Reconstr Surg. 2021;148(4):568e–80e.
15. Balaji SM. Burden of orofacial clefting in India, 2016: a global burden of disease approach. Ann Maxillofac Surg. 2018;8(1):91–100.

Chapter 2
The Cleft Care India Study 2019–2023: An Overview

Panchali Batra, Badri Thiruvenkatachari, Deborah Sybil, and Sakshi Katyal

2.1 Introduction

The Cleft Care India study (CCIS) is a project funded by the Ministry of Human Resources and Development (MHRD), now known as the Ministry of Education, under the Scheme for Promotion of Academic and Research Collaborations (SPARC). The project aimed at evaluating the standard of care of non-syndromic unilateral cleft lip and palate (UCLP) patients at ages 5, 12, and 20 across India. The investigating team consisted of investigators from India and the UK. The lead centres were from Jamia Millia Islamia and the University of Manchester, and Co-PIs from Safdarjung Hospital (Government tertiary care centre in Delhi), and the University of Sheffield. The goal of this inter-centre study was to assess the effectiveness of cleft care for Indian patients, with the ultimate goal of improving the services for patients with cleft in India. This book is a part of the CCIS project, which provides details of major cleft centres in India and facilities available, professionals and teams involved in cleft care, and academic activities at these centres. It

This book is a culmination of the CCIS project, which describes the journey of the paramount cleft centres across India to reach where they are today. The CCIS project served as an opportunity to join hands with prime cleft care centres in India which should result in wider opportunities for multicentric research collaboration and clinical trials in the future.

P. Batra (✉) · S. Katyal
Department of Orthodontics, Faculty of Dentistry, Jamia Millia Islamia, New Delhi, India
e-mail: p.batra@jmi.ac.in

B. Thiruvenkatachari
Research, Sree Balaji Dental College and Hospital, BIHER, Chennai, India

Orthodontics, University of Manchester, Manchester, UK

D. Sybil
Department of Oral Surgery, Faculty of Dentistry, Jamia Millia Islamia, New Delhi, India

P. Batra et al. (eds.), *The Cleft Care Framework in India*,
https://doi.org/10.1007/978-981-99-8968-3_2

also makes an effort to produce a register of services in India by mapping the paramount centres on the map of India which could be useful to patients and clinicians.

2.2 Background

It is estimated that around 35,000 children are born with orofacial clefts every year in India [1]. Cleft lip and/or palate is accompanied by a variety of dental and skeletal anomalies, causing a long-term impact on the patient's facial aesthetics, function, and self-esteem.

Many specialist services are required such as nursing, speech pathologists, audiologists, surgeons, dentists, orthodontists, psychologists, etc. for these patients. In India, majority of the surgical support is provided by external funding agencies like Smile Train, Akila Bhartha Mahila Seva Samaj (ABMSS), Operation Smile, etc. The rest of the cleft care services are being delivered in a fragmented way in India, with very few centres providing comprehensive care. The care for these patients is marked by controversies and multiple treatment protocols because of a lack of evidence-based research. Many international projects such as the Eurocleft study (1992) [2], the first in the league to analyse surgical outcomes in patients with unilateral cleft lip palate, followed by CSAG [3], American cleft [4], Netherlands (Dutchcleft) [5], and Scandinavian cleft [6] studies have been carried out in an effort to produce evidence and hence improve cleft care. In India, the Indicleft task force project (https://indicleft.icmr.org.in/home.html) was the first multi-centre project that evaluated the patterns of congenital orofacial birth defects, risk factors, and protocols of treatment given to patients with cleft [7].

The approach to cleft care can be a centralized model or a decentralized model. Both systems have their pros and cons. The creation of a comprehensive cleft centre where holistic treatment can be rendered will take significant resources and many years of cooperative, determined effort in a country like India. Till then a decentralized model would perhaps be better suited to develop a community-based network and referral system. This would create an interdisciplinary skilled team, equip the primary health care centres with skills for supportive care of CLP patients, educate the community, and create awareness regarding cleft anomaly. Many centres in India are providing these services in isolation. This project evaluated the standard of care of unilateral cleft lip and palate patients across India by collecting patient data at 5, 12, and 20 years, from major cleft centres in India and then analysing the outcomes based on standardized parameters.

2.3 Subjects and Methods

A cross-sectional cohort study design with prospective data collection adhering to the pre-set guidelines of record collection was formulated. Major cleft centres across India, either from government organizations or from external funding agencies like Smile Train, Akila Bharatha Mahila Seva Samaja (ABMSS), and Operation Smile were contacted via E-mails or telephonically or in national cleft conferences. The centres willing to participate were registered in a portal specifically developed for this project (http://www.ccis.org.in/). Each cleft care centre was targeted to submit thirty case records with UCLP on the web portal. This study was formulated using a Eurocleft study as a model to standardize the outcomes for easy comparisons in the Indian population. Fourteen cleft care centres contributed data on patients with unilateral cleft lip and plate. The list of centres that participated in the study is provided in Table 2.1 and diagrammatically presented in Fig. 2.1.

Table 2.1 Names of the Centres that participated in CCIS

S.No	Cleft Care Centres
1.	Sri Balaji Medical and Dental College & Hospital, Chennai, Tamil Nadu
2.	GSR Institute of Craniofacial and Plastic Surgery, Hyderabad, Telangana
3.	G S Memorial Plastic Surgery Hospital and Trauma Center, Uttar Pradesh
4.	Bhagwan Mahaveer Jain Hospital, Bengaluru, Karnataka
5.	All India Institute of Medical Sciences, Jodhpur
6.	Ashwini Hospital, Odisha
7.	Sant Parmanand Hospital, New Delhi
8.	JSS Dental College & Hospital, Mysuru, Karnataka
9.	Toothbuddies- BSTC, Telangana
10.	Amandeep Hospital, Amritsar, Punjab
11.	Sharad Pawar Dental College and Hospital, Wardha, Maharashtra
12.	INGA Health Foundation, Bengaluru, Karnataka
13.	Vivekananda Polyclinic and Institute of Medical Sciences, Lucknow, Uttar Pradesh
14.	Center For Craniofacial Anomalies, Yenopoya Dental College, Karnataka

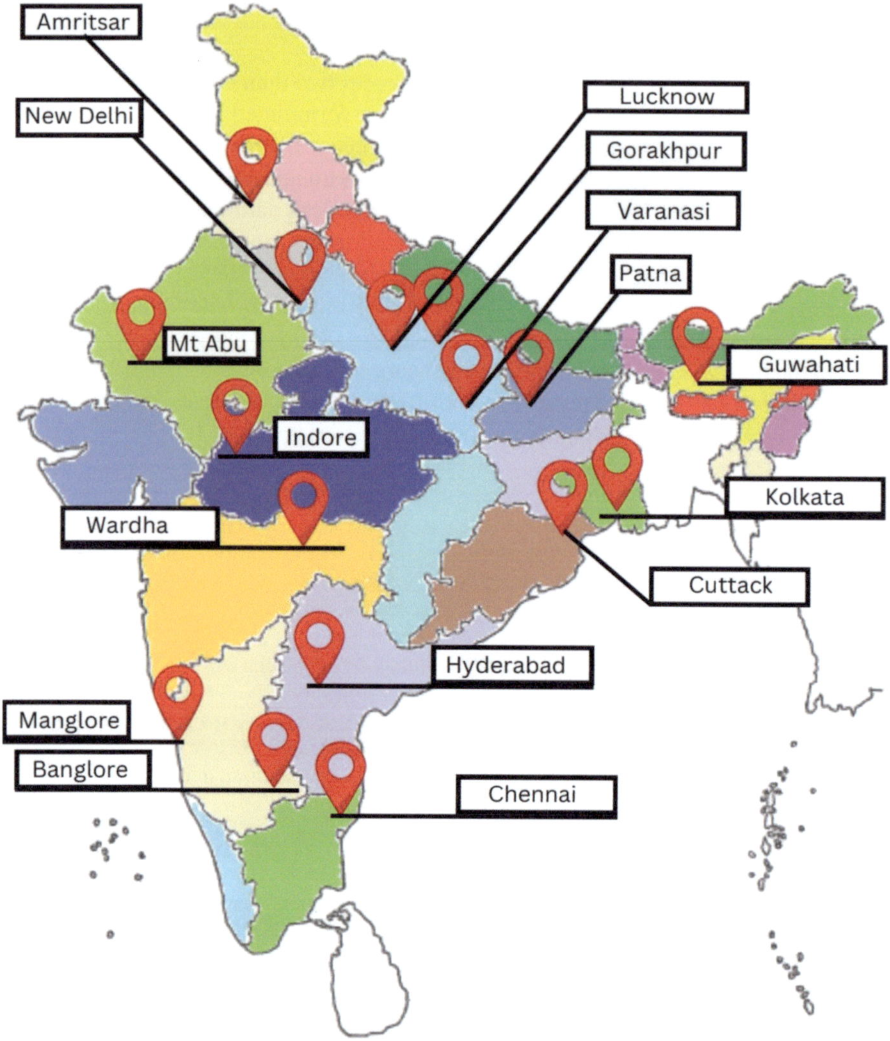

Fig. 2.1 Diagrammatic representation of PAN India participation of Cleft centres in CCIS

2.4 Study Population

The study included non-syndromic unilateral cleft lip and palate patients in the age groups of 5, 12, and 20 years. The age of the patients had to be within ± 6 months of the specified age group at the time when he reported in the centres. The specific age groups of 5, 12, and 20 were recorded since at 5 years, the surgical outcomes can best be evaluated, as no orthodontic intervention would have occurred at this age. At 12 years, the result of alveolar grafting procedures can be evaluated, and at 20 usually all interventions are complete.

2.5 Methodology

One clinician from each centre was trained during a workshop held in Dec 2019 at Jamia Millia Islamia by Dr. 1 Jonathan Sandy from the University of Bristol and Dr. Badri Thiruvenkatachari from the University of Manchester. An MOU was signed with the centres for data collection and execution of the project. For those centres that could not attend the workshop, online training sessions were conducted. The speech training was conducted by Savitha VH and Mr. Subramanian from Sri Ramachandra University. Voice recorders and speech samples of different languages were provided to the centre. The centres were supported with consumables or manpower for the smooth conduct of the project. The following records were taken of any UCLP patient who reported to the centre and was in the specified age group: Intraoral and extraoral photographs, study models, Radiographs (Lateral Cephalogram, OPG, Anterior oblique), Surgical Details form, Oral Health form, speech form, voice recordings, Intelligibility in context scale (ICS), and audiology form.

2.6 Discussion

Inter-centre comparisons have led to improvement in the quality of treatment provided to patients with cleft and also helped in abolishing unsafe practices. The success of this project relied on the willingness and commitment of the individual cleft team. It required vigorous training and calibration of the clinician responsible for taking records. All the centres followed the same protocols which led to standardized data collection.

This project could take possible future directions in the form of audits for various centres, multicentric research with these centres, and the integration or comparison with Eurocleft or Americleft. However, to evaluate the long-term intercentre outcomes, it is essential that dedicated manpower be appointed for data collection. The biggest challenge experienced in the project was the unwillingness of the teams due to a lack of research interest. Despite offering support in all forms, many centres did not join the project due to varied reasons.

The investigators very strongly feel that if a consensus is established amongst centres, to submit their data for evaluation, without any preconceived notions, India can be a forerunner in establishing standard operating procedures (SOP's) for cleft care.

References

1. Mossey P, Little J. Addressing the challenges of cleft lip and palate research in India. Indian J Plast Surg. 2009;42(Suppl):S9–18.
2. Shaw WC, Asher-McDade C, Brattström V, Dahl E, McWilliam J, Mølsted K, et al. A six-centre international study of treatment outcome in patients with clefts of the lip and palate: part 1. Principles and study design. Cleft Palate Craniofac J. 1992;29(5):393–7.
3. Sandy J, Williams A, Mildinhall S, Murphy T, Bearn D, Shaw B, et al. The Clinical Standards Advisory Group (CSAG) cleft lip and palate study. Br J Orthod. 1998;25(1):21–30.
4. Long RE, Hathaway R, Daskalogiannakis J, Mercado A, Russell K, Cohen M, et al. The Americleft study: an inter-centre study of treatment outcomes for patients with unilateral cleft lip and palate part 1. Principles and study design. Cleft Palate Craniofac J. 2011;48(3):239–43.
5. Prahl C, Kuijpers-Jagtman AM, Van't Hof MA, Prahl-Andersen B. A randomized prospective clinical trial of the effect of infant orthopaedics in unilateral cleft lip and palate: prevention of collapse of the alveolar segments (Dutchcleft). Cleft Palate Craniofac J. 2003;40(4):337–42.
6. Semb G, Enemark H, Friede H, Paulin G, Lilja J, Rautio J, et al. A Scandcleft randomised trials of primary surgery for unilateral cleft lip and palate: 1. Planning and management. J Plast Surg Hand Surg. 2017;51(1):2–13.
7. Kharbanda OP, Agrawal K, Khazanchi R, Sharma SC, Sagar S, Singhal M, et al. Clinical profile and treatment status of subjects with cleft lip and palate anomaly in India: preliminary report of a three-centre study. J Cleft Lip Palate Craniof Anomal. 2014;1(1):26.

Part II
The North India Experience

Chapter 3
Sant Parmanand Hospital, New Delhi

S. C. Söod, Puneet Batra, and Chetna Khandelwal

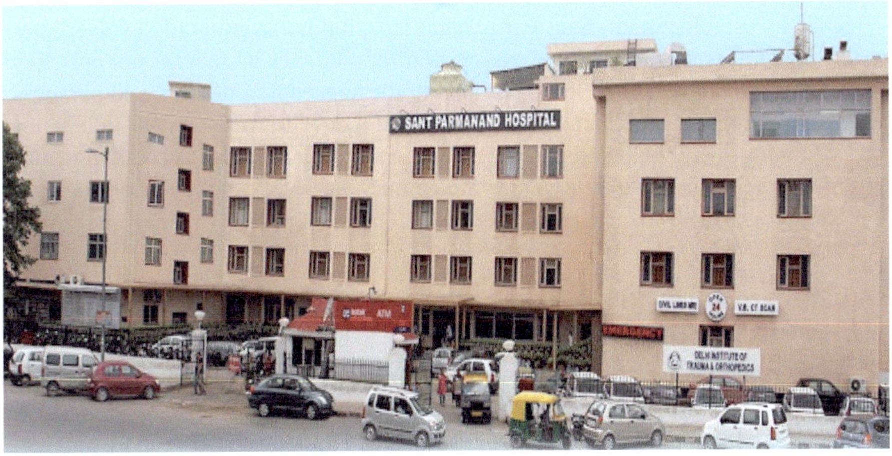

3.1 History of the Center

Sant Parmanand Hospital, established on 23rd February 2008, has made significant strides since its inception. Under the guidance of its pioneer, Sundereshwer Chander Sood, the hospital has become a renowned healthcare facility in Delhi. Dr. S C Sood, a highly respected member of the medical community, holds an impressive academic background, having obtained an MBBS from KGMC, Lucknow in 1985, followed by an MS in General Surgery and an MCh in Plastic Surgery from the same institution in 1988 and 1990, respectively. With over 32 years of experience in the field, Dr. S C Sood has been an invaluable asset to the center.

S. C. Söod · P. Batra (✉) · C. Khandelwal
Sant Parmanand Hospital, New Delhi, India

P. Batra et al. (eds.), *The Cleft Care Framework in India*,
https://doi.org/10.1007/978-981-99-8968-3_3

Throughout its history, the center has achieved several important milestones. In 2008, surgical interventions were introduced, with a remarkable 4,606 cases performed to date. Spearheaded by Dr. S C Sood, these interventions have played a crucial role in improving patient outcomes. In 2009, Prof Dr Puneet Batra joined the center and added the service of orthodontics, further expanding the range of treatments provided. Then, in 2015, Dr. Chetna Khandelwal became part of the team and introduced speech and language pathology services, enhancing the center's capabilities to address a wider range of patients. The center's commitment to excellence is further highlighted by its affiliation with Smile Train, one of the principal funding agencies. This partnership ensures that the center has access to necessary resources, enabling it to provide high-quality care to patients in need. Over the years, the hospital has also received support from secondary funding agencies, reinforcing its ability to deliver comprehensive medical services.

Since its establishment, Sant Parmanand Hospital has continually evolved, both in terms of infrastructure and the services it offers. It owes its success not only to its dedicated founder, Dr. S C Sood, but also to the succeeding doctors and personnel who have played key roles in shaping the center's development. With a rich history and a commitment to compassionate care, Sant Parmanand Hospital remains a prominent healthcare institution, striving to meet the evolving healthcare needs of the community it serves.

3.2 Present Scenario of the Center

Dr. Sagar Rajagopal is the Center Head of the medical facility. Alongside him, the center has a dedicated team of doctors, surgeons, clinicians, and support staff who contribute to the successful operation of the center. The doctors in the team include Dr. Sundereshwer Chander Sood, Dr. Pankaj Sharma, and Dr. Puneet Batra. The support staff consists of Chetna Khandelwal, Shalini Singh, Kanhaiya Singh, Jitendra, and others.

The center has performed a substantial number of surgeries over the years, with a total of 4606 cases operated on to date. To meet the needs of the patients, the center provides a wide range of services. Lip surgery, palate surgery, alveolar bone grafting, fistula closure, palate lengthening, VPI correction, orthognathic surgery, cleft rhinoplasty, and distraction osteogenesis are among the surgical procedures offered. Speech therapy, audiometry, orthodontics, nasoalveolar molding, general dentistry, nutritional services, psychiatric counseling, and ENT services (Grommet) are all available at the center. Dental radiography, computed tomography, 2D echocardiography, nasoendoscopy, and videofluoroscopy are among the diagnostic services provided by the center.

3.3 Workflow

The workflow system at the center follows a comprehensive approach. Upon referral, newborns are initially examined by the Orthodontist for PSIO if required. After this, the case is reviewed in the joint clinic and then planned for Lip repair in consultation with nutritionist, pediatrician, and anesthetists. Lip surgery is usually done at the age of 4–5 months. Palate repair is done at 9–12 months. Speech therapy is focused in the age group of 2–5 years. In the mixed dentition, patient is orthodontically treated to prepare for bone graft and maxillary protraction if indicated. Comprehensive orthodontics is done after permanent dentition has erupted. Some of the patients are operated for orthognathic surgery after cessation of growth with the help of orthodontics.

Despite their success, the center faces several challenges. Inadequate funding poses a significant obstacle, making it difficult to meet the growing demands and maintain high-quality services. The center also experiences challenges related to the stability of doctors, clinicians, and support staff, which may affect the continuity of patient care. Managing patient flow efficiently is another concern for the center. Additionally, patient follow-up presents a challenge, requiring dedicated efforts to ensure comprehensive care and monitoring beyond the initial treatment. Overcoming these challenges will enable the center to continue providing excellent care to their patients.

3.4 Clinical Protocol

The preferred surgical techniques for at the center are Modified Millards repair for lip correction and Furlows repair with primary buccal flaps for palate repair.

For primary surgeries, the average duration of admission for a patient at our center is typically 2–3 days. This duration may vary depending on the specific requirements and the progress of the patient's recovery. In the case of lip surgery, suture removal is typically scheduled after 7 days. This allows sufficient time for the wound to heal and ensures proper closure. For cleft palate patients, the center has a follow-up period of 4 weeks, during which their recovery is closely monitored. On the other hand, cleft lip patients are typically followed up for 10 days to ensure proper healing and address any concerns. Additionally, patients who are nutritionally deficient or anemic are scheduled for monthly follow-ups to assess their nutritional status and provide necessary interventions. Apart from these specific cases, regular appointments are scheduled based on the individual treatment protocol devised for each patient.

Patient and attender accommodation, transport allowance, food services, rehabilitation services are all offered by the center.

3.5 Community Outreach

This center focuses on serving the National Capital Region and reaches out to needy patients through various means. Referrals from primary healthcare centers enable this center to identify patients who require specialized services. Cleft camps are also conducted by the center. The center's popularity through word of mouth has also been instrumental in reaching out to those who require their services. Moreover, they actively engage in door-to-door campaigns in slums and rural areas, where their team visits communities to raise awareness about cleft lip and palate and provide information about their services and available treatments.

3.6 Academic and Research Activities

One of the notable achievements is the development of Aligner NAM, a revolutionary technique that has been successfully implemented at the center. The effectiveness of Aligner NAM has been widely recognized, leading to its adoption and initiation in numerous centers around the world.

3.7 Future Direction

The center aims to expand the comprehensive care specialists and aims to be a leader in research and innovation. To the next generation of cleft care personnel, the center emphasizes the importance of hard work and patience in achieving success in this specialized field. Cleft care requires a multidisciplinary approach and future centers should adopt the principles of TEAM Work and CCC (Comprehensive Cleft Care). By fostering collaboration among various specialists, including surgeons, orthodontists, speech therapists, psychologists, and social workers, holistic care for every patient can be ensured. In the context of cleft care in India, the lack of comprehensive cleft care teams has been a significant challenge. However, the landscape is evolving, and we are witnessing a positive change with the increasing number of dedicated specialists committed to providing comprehensive cleft care. Through continued efforts, there is a hope to bridge this gap and ensure that every individual with a cleft condition receives the best possible care and support.

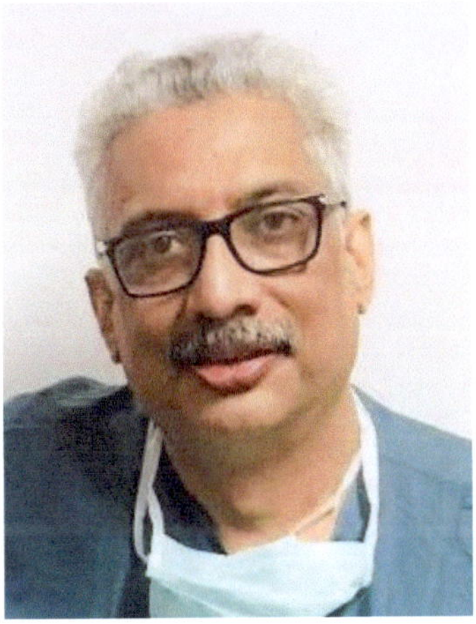

Dr. S C Sood (Plastic Surgeon)

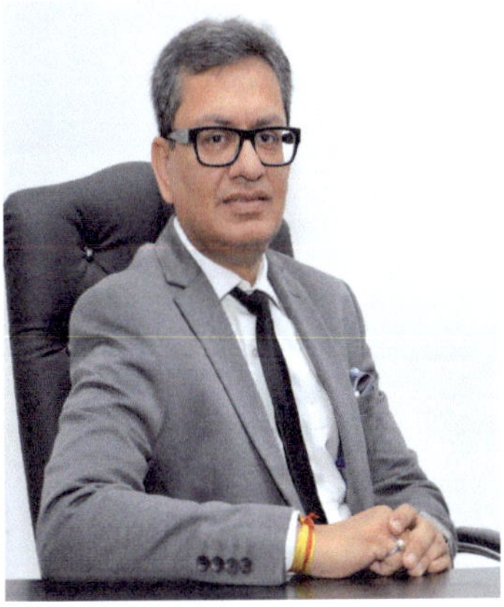

Dr. Puneet Batra (Orthodontist)

Chapter 4
Vivekananda Poly Clinic and Research Institute, Lucknow, Uttar Pradesh

Panchali Batra and Kamlesh Singh

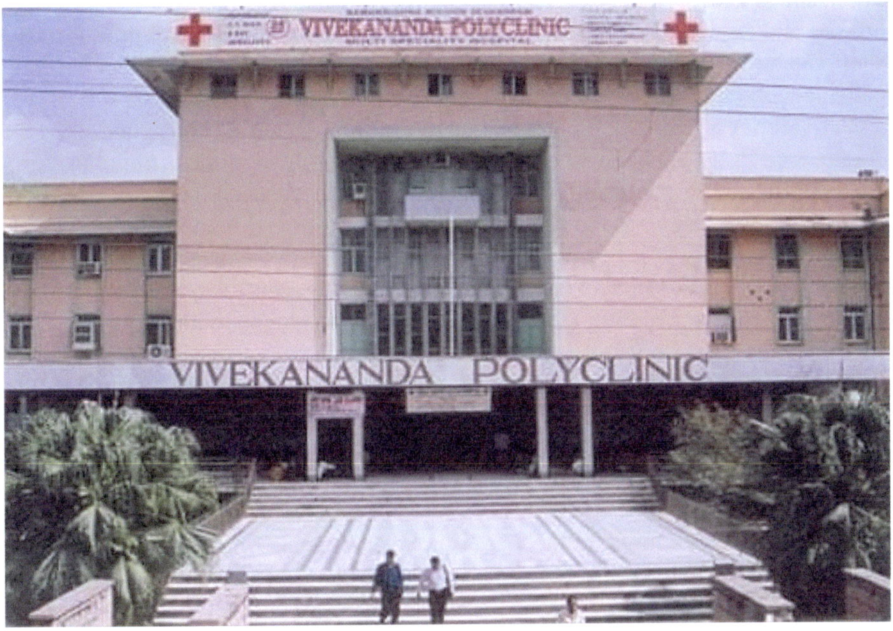

P. Batra (✉)
Department of Orthodontics, Faculty of Dentistry, Jamia Millia Islamia, New Delhi, India
e-mail: p.batra@jmi.ac.in

K. Singh
Department of Orthodontics and Dentofacial Orthopaedics, Saraswati Dental College and Hospital, Lucknow, UP, India

Vivekananda Polytechnic and Institute of Medical Sciences, Lucknow, UP, India

P. Batra et al. (eds.), *The Cleft Care Framework in India*,
https://doi.org/10.1007/978-981-99-8968-3_4

4.1 History of the Center

The Smile Train Project, Vivekananda Poly Clinic and Research Institute in Lucknow, with its address at 226007, was established in February 2005.

The center has reached several key milestones since its start. Cleft lip and palate surgeries could be made possible through the collaboration between Smile Train and VPIMS Lucknow in 2005. The center's commitment to comprehensive care led to the introduction of cleft lip and palate orthodontics in 2009, followed by cleft lip and palate speech therapy in 2010, all facilitated by the partnership between Smile Train and VPIMS Lucknow. These expansions enhanced the scope of services offered and provided holistic care to patients. In 2022, the center introduced the Cleft Lip and Palate Nutrition Program, aiming to address the nutritional needs of patients with cleft lip and palate.

Dr. Vaibhav Khanna (Craniofacial surgeon), the pioneer of the center, played a crucial role in its establishment and development. Following his efforts, Dr. Amit Agarwal (plastic surgeon) and other personnel have succeeded him and continued to contribute significantly to the center's growth. The principal funding agency for the center is the Smile Train Project USA, while VPIMS (Vivekanand polyclinic and institute of medical sciences), Lucknow serves as the secondary funding agency, enabling the center to continue its valuable work in serving individuals with cleft lip and palate.

4.2 Present Scenario of the Center

The capable steering force for the team is none other than Dr. Amit Agarwal serving as Center head; augmenting his skills is an admirable group including Dr. Richa Srivastava, Dr. Kamlesh Singh, Dr. Himanshu Trivedi alongside Dr. Neeta Bhargava, and Dr. Harshita Srivastava combined with dynamic personnel, Mrs. Payal Mukhi Ahuja, Mr. Anees Prajapati, Mr. Neeraj Singh, Mr. Neeraj Yadav, and Mr. Hariom.

The center has operated on approximately 9000 cases so far which demonstrates their expertise and experience in the field.

The center offers a wide range of services to cater to the needs of the patients. In terms of surgical services, it provides treatments such as lip surgery, palate surgery, alveolar bone grafting, fistula closure, palate lengthening, VPI correction, orthognathic surgery, cleft rhinoplasty, and distraction osteogenesis. Additionally, the center provides rehabilitation services, including speech therapy, audiometry, orthodontics, nasoalveolar molding, general dentistry, nutritionist services, and ENT services for grommet insertion. Diagnostic services which are available here include dental radiography, computed tomography, 2D echocardiography, and nasoendoscopy.

4.3 Workflow System

The center has implemented a well-organized workflow system to effectively manage and correct cleft anomalies and prioritizes a team approach to ensure comprehensive care for the patients. The process begins with the involvement of a Plastic/Cranio Facial surgeon who is responsible for diagnosing the condition and performing the necessary surgical treatments. A pediatrician plays a vital role in the well-being of the patients, nutritional care, and pre-anesthetic evaluations. An orthodontist is involved in the treatment of teeth and jaw abnormalities, working closely with the surgeon to coordinate the overall treatment plan. The center has a speech therapist who conducts comprehensive speech evaluations, provides therapy, and monitors the progress of the patients throughout their developmental stages. An ENT Specialist is also in the team and is in charge of diagnosing and managing any ear infections or hearing loss issues, as well as a Nursing Coordinator, who not only delivers nutrition packets but also counsels families about their nutritional needs, ensuring they understand and follow the necessary guidelines.

The center does face several challenges. Inadequate funding poses a significant obstacle. The instability of doctors and clinicians is another challenge the center encounters, which can disrupt the continuity of care for the patients. Similarly, the instability of support staff also affects the smooth functioning of the center. Patient flow is yet another challenge which the center faces. The lack of funding specifically allocated for comprehensive dental care limits the addressal of dental issues related to cleft anomalies effectively.

4.4 Clinical Protocol

The preferred surgical techniques for lip and palate correction at the center include rotation/advancement and its variants (MILLARD), straight line repair (FISCHER), BLACK Procedure, VY procedure, and Bardach's procedure, each with their own specific approaches and modifications for effective correction.

For primary surgeries, the average length of admission for patients is approximately 1 week. After the primary lip surgery, suture removal typically takes place after 1 week. Patients are scheduled for regular appointments to monitor their healing progress and if a patient misses an appointment, the center contacts them by phone to reschedule the appointment and provide the required support.

Patient and attender accommodation, transport allowance, food services, and rehabilitation services are all available at the center.

4.5 Community Outreach

The center is dedicated to community outreach and providing healthcare services to individuals in Uttar Pradesh, Bihar, and Nepal and has employed various methods to reach out to those in need. The center receives referrals from primary health care centers which helps to extend services to patients who require specialized treatment. The center organizes cleft camps and word of mouth has also played a significant role in the center's popularity. Furthermore, social media platforms are used to raise awareness about the services and connect with a wider audience. The center collaborates with government agencies and primary health centers to offer free eye surgeries and provide medical treatment for patients below the poverty line.

4.6 Academic and Research Activities

Over the years, the center has successfully carried out more than ten research activities. The center's mission has been to provide comprehensive cleft care to the disadvantaged community, delivering free services that cover a wide range of treatments and procedures.

4.7 Future Direction

The future vision of this center is to establish and maintain a standard of excellence in providing quality comprehensive cleft care. It strives to ensure that individuals with cleft lip and palate receive the best possible treatment, encompassing all aspects of their care from infancy to adulthood. The goal is to improve their overall quality of life and enable them to fully integrate into society. To the next generation of cleft care personnel, the center emphasizes the privilege of being associated with cleft care and encourages them to seek training from reputed centers. For future cleft centers, the center recommends prioritizing comprehensive cleft care, addressing all the physical, emotional, and social needs of patients. Finally, in India, cleft care lacks adequate funding and training for the cleft care team. It is crucial to invest in resources and education to bridge these gaps and ensure that every individual with a cleft receives the care they deserve.

4 Vivekananda Poly Clinic and Research Institute, Lucknow, Uttar Pradesh

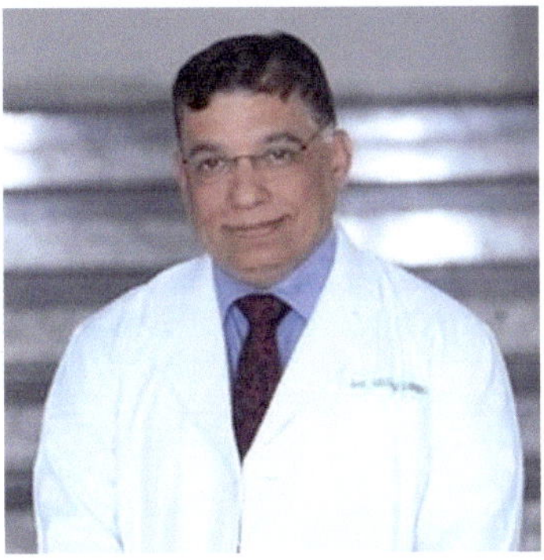

Dr. Vaibhav Khanna (Plastic surgeon)

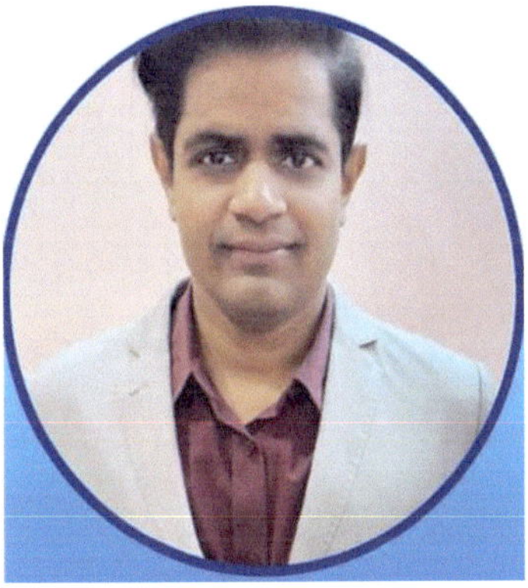

Dr. Amit Agarwal (Plastic surgeon)

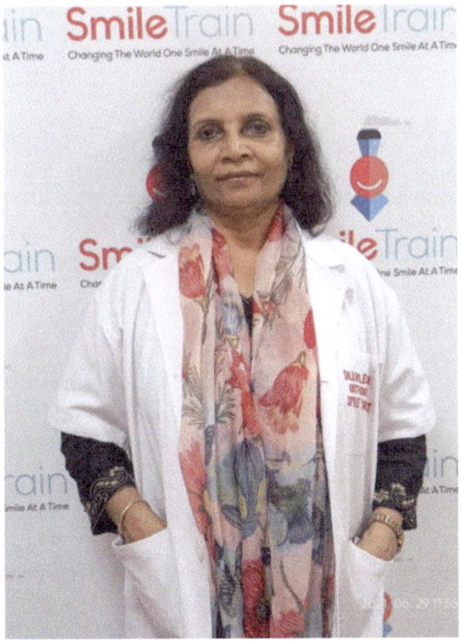

Dr. Kamlesh Singh (Orthodontist)

Chapter 5
Amandeep Hospital, Amritsar, Punjab

Deborah Sybil, Ravi K. Mahajan, Sukhdeep Singh Kahlon, Abhishek Bhamre, Krishnan Srinivasan, Adish Jain, and Samiksha Chopra

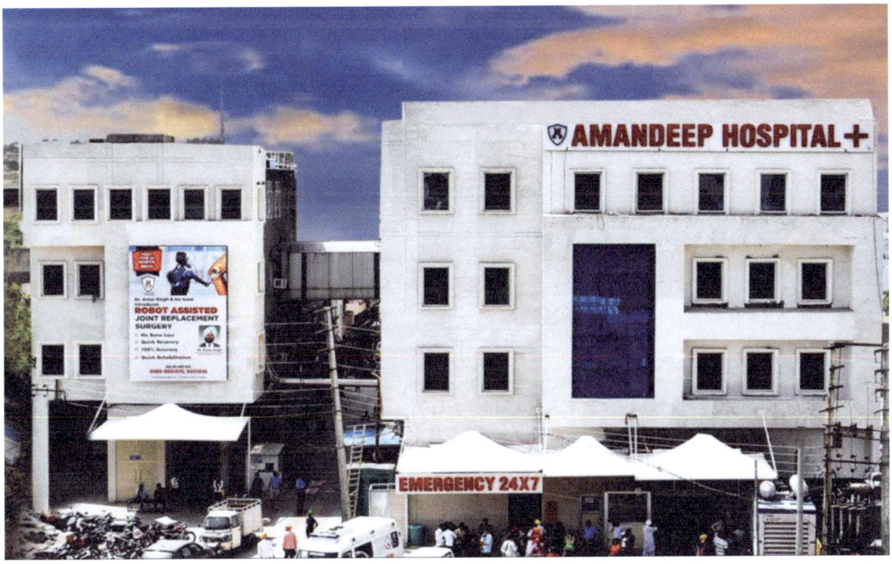

5.1 History of the Center

Amandeep Hospital, located in Amritsar, began its journey in September 2004 and has since then reached multiple significant milestones. The center has continually strived to improve its services and infrastructure. In 2010, Amandeep Hospital established a dedicated Smile Train Ward. The center started providing Orthognathic

D. Sybil (✉)
Department of Oral Surgery, Faculty of Dentistry, Jamia Millia Islamia, New Delhi, India

R. K. Mahajan · S. S. Kahlon · A. Bhamre · K. Srinivasan · A. Jain · S. Chopra
Smile Train Centre, Amandeep Hospital, Amritsar, India

P. Batra et al. (eds.), *The Cleft Care Framework in India*,
https://doi.org/10.1007/978-981-99-8968-3_5

Surgery Services, led by Dr. Ravi Kumar Mahajan and Dr. S. S. Kahlon from the year 2013. In 2016, nasoendoscopy was introduced, fore-fronted by Dr. Adish Jain, at the hospital for evaluations of VPI patients. The hospital introduced an in-house daily Orthodontic Clinic in 2018, with Dr. S. S. Kahlon, Dr. Samiksha Chopra, and Dr. Manmeet Kaur Bagga leading the service. The same year also saw the establishment of an in-house daily speech therapy center, under the guidance of Dr. Jyoti and Dr. Ravi Shankar, which is presently headed by Dr. Renuka Sharma. Dr. Ravi Kumar Mahajan who is the chief plastic surgeon and also the pioneer of plastic surgery services at this hospital serves as the Director, Smile Train Project.

The center owes its success to the talented doctors and personnel who have contributed enormously to its growth. Notable individuals include Dr. Ravi Kumar Mahajan, Dr. Abhishek Bhamre, Dr. Krishnan Srinivasan, Dr. Adish Jain, Dr. Paryesh Gupta, Dr. Harish Ghildyal, Dr. Krishna Prasad Prusty, and Dr. S. Mahipal Singh, all of whom serve as Consultant Plastic Surgeons. Dr. S. S. Kahlon heads the Orthodontic department, with the support of Dr. Samiksha Chopra and Dr. Manmeet Kaur Bagga, who work as Consultant Orthodontists. Dr. S. S. Kahlon has been providing orthodontic services to cleft patients since 2004 when Smile Train Project was started at Amandeep Hospital. The Center's Speech Pathology services were started in the beginning by Dr. Sanjay Kumar and later overseen by Dr. Ravi Shankar, Dr. Neha Solanki, and Dr. Jyoti. The team of anesthesiologists comprises Dr. Monica Sarad, Dr. Sunil Dutt, Dr. Bhawna Madan, Dr. R. P. Singh, Dr. Ravi Kant Sharma, and Dr. Pankaj Soni.

Amandeep Hospital has grown as a premier healthcare institution, delivering exceptional plastic surgery, orthodontic, speech therapy, and anesthesia services to the community, thanks to the joint efforts of devoted medical professionals and the help of its funding agency, The Smile Train.

5.2 Present Scenario of the Center

The doctors, surgeons, clinicians, support staff, and team consist of plastic surgeons including Dr. Mahajan, Dr. Abhishek Bhamre, Dr. Krishnan Srinivasan, and Dr. Adish Jain and Dr. Tarun Chaudhary, Dr. Amreen Kaur, oral and maxillofacial surgeon, are also part of the cleft surgery team. Dr. S. S. Kahlon and Dr. Samiksha Chopra are the orthodontists and Dr. Jyoti is the speech therapist. Dr. Monica Sarad, Dr. Sunil Dutt, Dr. Bhawna Madan, and Dr. R. P. singh form the anesthesiologist's team while Dr. Amandeep Kaur and Dr. Jasleen Kaur are the pediatricians.

The support staff include Mr. Dalbir Singh, the Smile Train Coordinator, Mr. Karan, a counselor, Ms. Rajwinder Kaur, the OPD Supervisor, Ms. Baljeet Kaur, Mr. Ramanjit Singh, Ms. Parminder Kaur, Ms. Navdeep Kaur, Mr. Varinder Singh, and Mr. Sarabjit Singh who all serve as OT Technicians.

The center has a remarkable track record, having successfully treated 8000 cases to date. Lip surgery, palate surgery, alveolar bone grafting, fistula closure, palate lengthening, VPI correction, orthognathic surgery, cleft rhinoplasty, and distraction osteogenesis are among the surgical services provided. Except for orthognathic surgery and distraction osteogenesis, which started in 2013, these surgical treatments have been performed since 2004.

The hospital offers rehabilitation services in addition to surgeries. Speech therapy, orthodontics, nasoalveolar molding, and psychological assistance are among them. In 2004, the center began offering speech therapy and, the following year, orthodontics and nasoalveolar molding. In order to provide complete care to patients, a psychologist was recently recruited to the team in 2022. Furthermore, the center has had a dedicated counselor since 2015 to support patients and their families.

The center also offers diagnostic services, including dental radiography since 2004, 2D echocardiography since 2017 and nasoendoscopy since 2016.

5.3 Workflow System

To ensure effective patient care and treatment, the center has a well-organized workflow system. The process starts with the patient visiting the OPD with a free consultation slip. The patient undergoes a consultation with a surgeon to assess their condition. Depending on the case, a cross consultation may be arranged with an orthodontist or speech therapist for further evaluation. Routine investigations are then conducted to gather necessary diagnostic information followed by pediatric consultation. PAC is carried out by an anesthesiologist to evaluate the patient's fitness for surgery. Counseling sessions are conducted by a dedicated counselor. The patients are admitted under the Smile Train project and are subsequently shifted to the dedicated Smile Train ward. The surgeon and anesthesiologist conduct a same-day ward round and the required surgical procedure is carried out in the OT. Patients are discharged 2–3 days after surgery but those coming from far off areas may be admitted to the hospital until the sutures are removed. Regular follow-up appointments are arranged based on the type of surgery performed and the need for additional therapy.

One of the primary challenges the center faces is the instability of support staff, which can affect the smooth functioning of the workflow system. Another problem the center has been facing is the non-availability of a regular speech therapist, which can impact the timely evaluation and treatment of patients requiring speech-related interventions.

5.4 Clinical Protocol

Modified Millard's Technique is used for lip repair, and Modified Langenbeck Technique is utilized for palate repair at the center and a patient needs to be admitted for a period of 3–6 days for primary surgeries. Sutures in a lip surgery are removed after 6 days. The patients are called for regular follow-up keeping in mind the distance from where patient is coming. Counselor stays in touch with all patients.

The center has provision for accommodation, transport allowance, food services, rehabilitation services for the patients and their attenders.

5.5 Community Outreach

This center has an extensive area of reach, covering all the border districts of Punjab, the entire Jammu and Kashmir region, and parts of Haryana, Himachal Pradesh, and Rajasthan. This ensures that the center reaches out to a large population and provides support to those in need. Referrals from primary health care centers, cleft camps, the center's popularity (word of mouth), and the distribution of posters and pamphlets to every discharged patient to raise awareness of this project in their respective areas are some of the ways through which this center has reached out to needy patients.

5.6 Academic and Research Activities

The center has had several cleft fellowships, training a number of talented individuals who have made notable achievements in the field of oral and maxillofacial surgery. Dr. Rahul Chhajlani, Dr. Gogulanathan, Dr. Ankit Khasgiwala, Dr. Amreen Kaur, and Dr. Kunal Gupta, all MDS in Oral and Maxillofacial Surgery, have received training at the center.

The center has been involved in various funded research projects and scientific publications. Noteworthy research papers include "Macroglossia following palatoplasty causing upper airway obstruction: Case report" by Ruchi Gupta et al., published in the Journal of Oral and Maxillofacial Surgery in 2001. Additionally, Ravi Mahajan et al. have published several papers, such as "Evaluation of Secondary and Late Secondary Alveolar Bone Grafting on 66 Unilateral Cleft Lip and Palate Repair" (2017), "Nasopharyngeal Dermoids and Cleft Palate" (2018) in the American Cleft Palate-Craniofacial Association, and "A retrospective analysis of incidence and management of palatal fistula" (2019) in the Indian Journal of Plastic Surgery. Another notable contribution by Ravi Mahajan et al. is their research on the role of tongue flap in palatal fistula repair, which they presented in a series of 41 cases published in the Indian Journal of Plastic Surgery in 2019. Furthermore, the center is actively involved in the NAMUC (Nasoalveolar Molding in Unilateral Cleft) Study, conducted in collaboration with Balaji Dental College, Chennai.

The center's important contributions to cleft care extend beyond research and publications. They have been pioneers in their region, providing comprehensive cleft care to patients.

5.7 Future Direction

The future vision of the center is to further develop it as a center of excellence for comprehensive cleft care that not only provides surgical interventions but also focuses on holistic care, including pre-surgical evaluation, post-operative rehabilitation, orthodontic treatment, speech therapy, and psychological support. By integrating all these aspects into practice, it strives to enhance the quality of life for individuals with cleft lip and palate.

The center believes that comprehensive cleft care is a team work and every member of the team is important and should be given due regard.

Cleft care in India lacks a strong team approach, owing to a scarcity of cleft orthodontists and cleft speech pathologists. While qualified cleft surgeons and other specialists are involved in cleft treatment, the lack of specialized orthodontic and speech therapy knowledge impedes full management of cleft lip and palate.

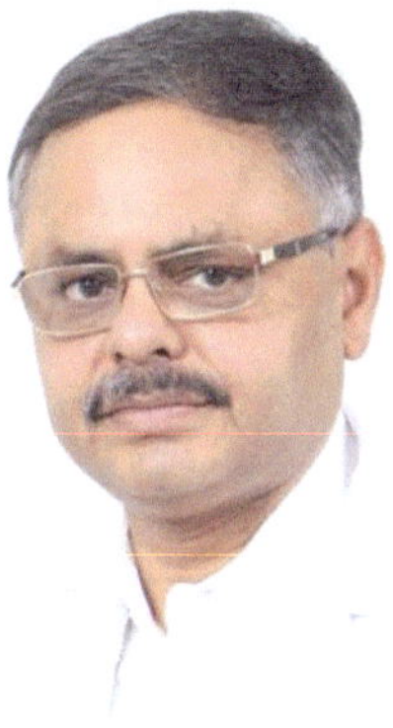

Dr. Ravi Kumar Mahajan (Plastic surgeon)

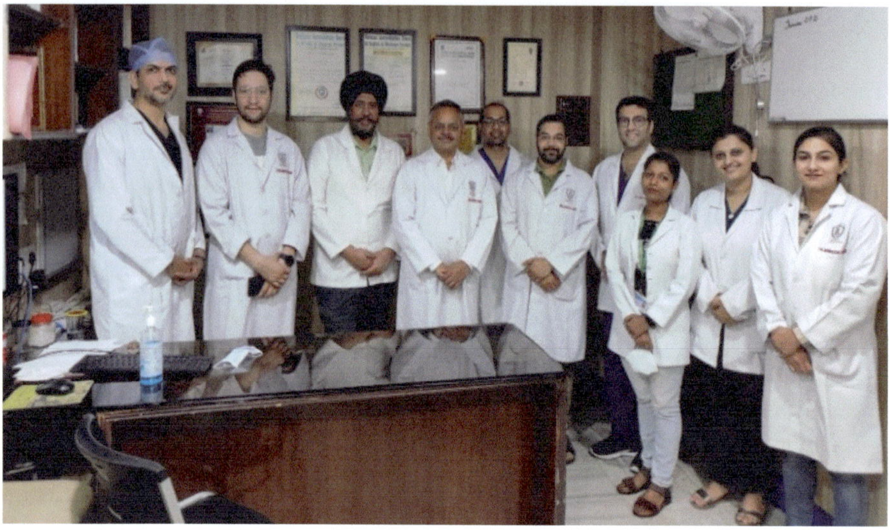

Smile Train Project Team From Left to Right - Dr. Krishnan Srinivasan, Dr. Samik Sharma, Dr. Sukhdeep Singh Kahlon, Dr. Ravi K Mahajan, Dr. Abhishek Bhamre, Dr. Adish Jain, Dr. Tarun Choudhary, Dr. Jyoti, Dr. Samiksha Chopra, Dr. Amreen Kaur

Chapter 6
Savitri Hospital and Research Centre, Gorakhpur, Uttar Pradesh

Badri Thiruvenkatachari and Asif Masood

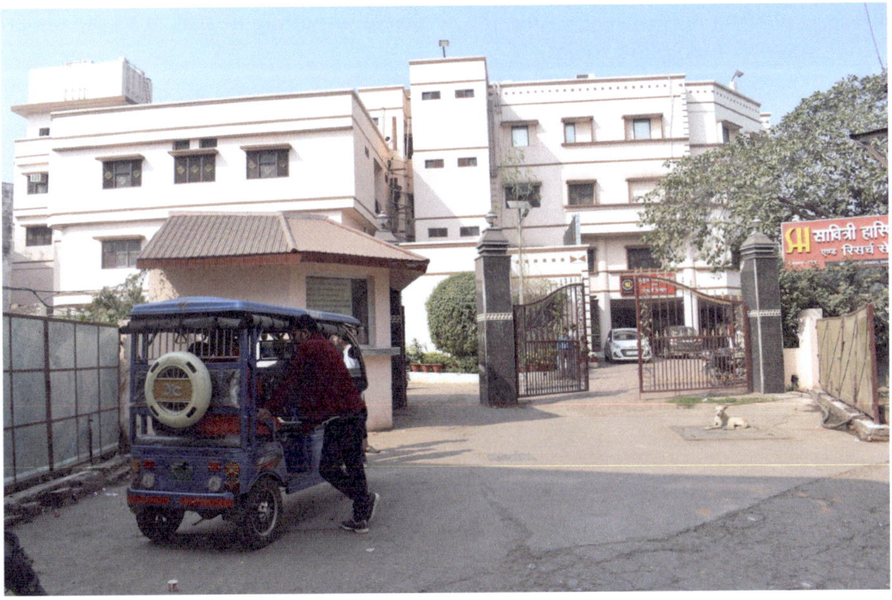

6.1 History of the Centre

The Savitri Hospital and Research Centre is a well-known cleft care centre. The Cleft Unit was started in September 2005 in partnership with Smile Train. The centre under the leadership of Dr. Asif Masood has managed to achieve great

---

B. Thiruvenkatachari (✉)
Dental Research, Sree Balaji Medical College and Hospital, The Cleft and Craniofacial Centre, Chennai, Tamil Nadu, India

A. Masood
Savitri Hospital and Research Centre, Dilezakpur, Gorakhpur, Uttar Pradesh, India

P. Batra et al. (eds.), *The Cleft Care Framework in India*,
https://doi.org/10.1007/978-981-99-8968-3_6

milestones over the years. The first year of the centre's inception saw the introduction of successful cleft lip and palate surgeries by Dr. Masood, giving hope to many patients. The addition of speech therapy services by Ms. Abha in 2012 marked another significant milestone expanding the centre's holistic care approach. Under the able guidance of Dr. Isha Jain Gulati, the centre expanded its services to include orthodontics in 2016. The centre also witnessed the introduction of VPI surgery, another achievement by Dr. Masood. The role of succeeding doctors and personnel along with Dr. Masood cannot be understated. Dr. Hassan Fareed, Dr. Rifat Hussain (Visiting surgeon USA), Dr. Isha Gulati, and Mr. Rafique Ahmad have immensely contributed towards the continued growth and success of the centre. Smile Train is the sole funding agency supporting the centre in providing treatment to the underprivileged sections of the society.

6.2 Present Scenario of the Centre

This centre has a devoted team of healthcare specialists who work day in and day out to provide comprehensive care to cleft lip and palate patients. Dr. Asif Masood, an experienced and highly qualified professional leads the centre along with Dr. Hassan Fareed (BDS), Dr. Isha Gulati MDS (Orthodontics), Mr. Rafique Ahmad, Ms. Shambhavi Pandey (Nutritionist), Dr. Maqsood Alam (Anaesthetist), and Dr. K. Siddiqui (Anaesthetist). The centre holds the distinction of operating more than 15,000 cases till date.

The centre offers surgical, rehabilitation, and diagnostic services to cater to specific patient needs. It specializes in lip surgery, palate surgery, alveolar bone grafting, fistula closure, palate lengthening, VPI correction, and cleft rhinoplasty. Various rehabilitation services that are currently available include speech therapy, orthodontics, nasoalveolar moulding, general dentistry, and nutrition counselling and support. Diagnostic services, namely, dental radiography, computed tomography, 2D echocardiography, and nasoendoscopy are also available at the centre.

6.3 Workflow

This centre is a high-volume cleft centre where cleft surgeries are being done from 1995 but the volumes picked up after partnership with Smile Train in 2005. Initially, cleft (Smile Train) surgeries were done at Star Hospital and it was subsequently moved to its current location at Savitri hospital in 2007.

Majority of the patients come to this centre from Eastern UP, Bihar, and Nepal. All patients are seen in the OPD, investigated accordingly and planned for surgery. Follow-up patients are seen by the surgeon and then referred to Speech/Orthodontics as required.

Though Smile Train is the only funding agency, the centre does not face challenges in this regard but does face certain issues like unavailability of trained clinicians and support staff.

6.4 Clinical Protocol

Millards Repair for lip, Furlows and Langenbecks repair for palate are the preferred techniques for correction at the centre. Patients are admitted for a duration of 2–3 days for primary surgeries. Suture removal is done after a week in lip surgeries. All patients irrespective of the type of surgery done are seen 1 week after discharge. The second visit commences 2-week post-surgery, while the third visit is scheduled after 1 month followed by the fourth visit after 3 months. Subsequent appointments are scheduled as per requirements.

The centre has a guest house for patient attendants, which is available at a very nominal price. Free transport facility is available for patients who cannot pay and dietary requirements of patients during hospital stay are well taken care of.

6.5 Community Outreach

The centre provides treatment to patients from eastern Uttar Pradesh, parts of Bihar and even Nepal. Various ways are employed to reach out to needy patients. The centre receives referrals from primary health care centres through RBSK(Rashtriya Bal Swasthya Karyakram). Additionally, there is a dedicated outreach team that covers rural areas, coordinating with RBSK to reach out to patients seeking treatment for cleft deformities. The centre has also reached larger community through word of mouth. Smile Train has a partnership with RBSK which helps to identify and bring patients to the centre.

6.6 Future Direction

The centre aims to continue providing free cleft services, achieving excellence in cleft care and envisions becoming a training centre for cleft care.

Cleft care is not mere correction of cleft lip and palate. It is the multi-speciality comprehensive cleft care which is the need of the hour. All cleft centres should strive to develop comprehensive cleft care units with adequate number of trained professionals. Smaller places often have problems with the availability of trained cleft care professionals. Although India has one of the largest proportions of cleft patients who are receiving treatment, but due to lack of publications and reporting the work being done in this regard is still not recognized. The excellent work that is being done here should find a place in publishing.

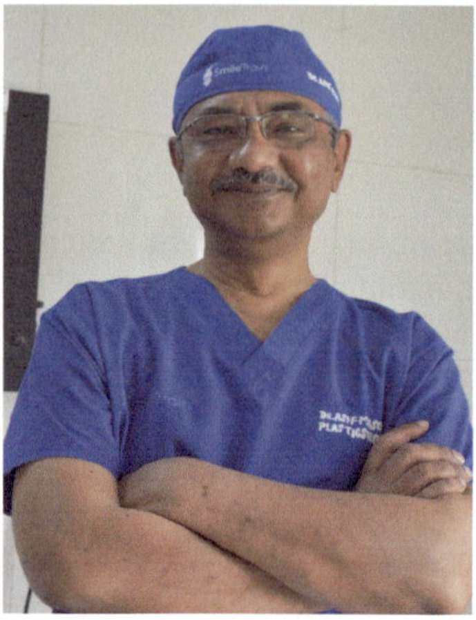

Dr. Asif Masood (Plastic Surgeon)

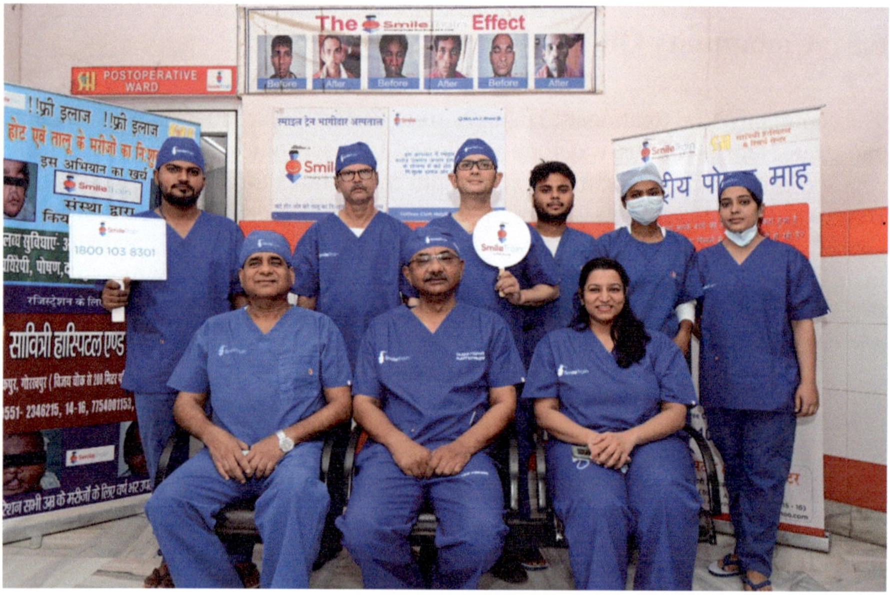

Cleft care team Sitting (L to R): Maqsood Alam (Anaesthetist), Asif Masood (Plastic Surgeon), Isha Jain (Orthodontist) Standing-Shahid Husain (Nursing Staff), Rashid Ali (Nursing Staff), Hassan Fareed (Dentist), Osama (Nursing Staff), Preeti (Nursing Staff), Shambhavi Pandey (Nursing Staff)

Chapter 7
G S Memorial Plastic Surgery Hospital, Varanasi, Uttar Pradesh

Deborah Sybil, Subodh Kumar Singh, and Ishan Singh

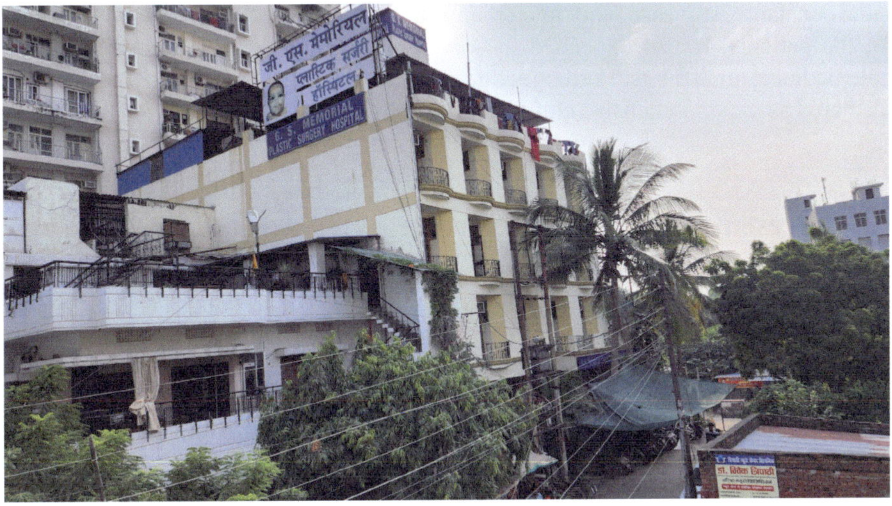

7.1 History of the Center

Right from its very inception in 2001, GS Memorial Plastic Surgery Hospital, Varanasi has a rich history of transformative accomplishments. The hospital has achieved quite significant milestones leaving an indelible impression in the field of plastic surgery. The hospital entered into a landmark collaboration with Smile Train on the 1st of April, 2004 which set the stage for trailblazing advancements. By the end of 2005, the hospital had successfully completed over 2500 primary cleft surgeries. This number increased to 8000 by the year 2008. The hospital completed

D. Sybil (✉)
Department of Oral Surgery, Faculty of Dentistry, Jamia Millia Islamia, New Delhi, India

S. K. Singh · I. Singh
G S Memorial Plastic Surgery Hospital, Varanasi, India

P. Batra et al. (eds.), *The Cleft Care Framework in India*,
https://doi.org/10.1007/978-981-99-8968-3_7

20,000 surgeries by May 2011 and reached a whopping number of 40,000 by June 2023. The hospital's impact of its work and methodology was heightened by the documentary, "Smile Pinki" which got international recognition and acclaim. This documentary earned the prestigious Academy Award (Oscar) in the Documentary Short Section in 2009. Pinki and Dr. Subodh were also invited to Wimbledon finals in 2013, where Pinki did the toss.

Apart from its surgical achievements, the hospital fosters a wide variety of in-house services catering to the holistic well-being of the patients. It started cleft genetic research with BHU in the year 2005. From the introduction of speech services in 2005, nutrition services in 2006 to Missed call campaign in 2009, the hospital constantly strives to work toward improvement of the experiences and outcomes of the patients. It also expanded its services to include orthodontic services and telemedicine in 2011 and orthognathic services in 2022. In the year 2023, it was declared as a comprehensive cleft care center by Smile Train.

7.2 Present Scenario of the Center

The center headed by Dr. Subodh Kumar Singh is a testament to exceptional cleft care.

Dr. Singh's legacy is being upheld by a succession of distinguished doctors, surgeons, clinicians, and support staff including Dr. K C Gupta, Dr. A N Singh, Dr. Gaurav Nayyar, Dr. Ishan Singh, Dr. Menka Pandey, Dr. Pratima Rathor, Dr. Prabhat Pathak, Dr. Abhinav Raj Gupta, Dr. Ansari, Mrs. Sapna Mishra, Mr. Pankaj Singh, Mr. Amit Srivastava, Mr. Nisar Ahmed, Mrs. Usha and Miss Shobha. Their combined efforts have led to a phenomenal record of operating 40,300 cases till date.

The center offers a range of services encompassing surgical, rehabilitation, and diagnostic domains. Surgical services include lip surgery, palate surgery, alveolar bone grafting, Fistula closure, palate lengthening, VPI correction, and cleft rhinoplasty since 2004, orthognathic surgery since 2022, and distraction osteogenesis since 2023. The rehabilitation services being offered include speech therapy, audiometry, and counselor services since 2005, nutritionist since 2006, ENT services (Grommet) since 2009, orthodontics since 2011, and naso-alveolar molding and general dentist since 2021 each. Diagnostic services like dental radiography and nasoendoscopy are also available.

WORKFLOW SYSTEM: The center has a robust outreach program for the last 19 years. Dedicated team of social workers spread information throughout the interiors of all districts in neighboring states. Patients are registered in screening camps and also walk into the hospital. The patients are thoroughly evaluated by the nutritionists, surgeon, pediatrician, and anesthesiologist and are fully investigated. A treatment plan is developed, and surgeries and other services are provided as required. Patients are kept in regular follow-up by center visit, telemedicine as well as home visits. Patients get timely nutrition advice, surgeries, speech, oral health, and orthodontic care. In-house orthognathic surgeries are also available. The center is funded by Smile train.

Despite its accomplishments, the center faces challenges including the need for increased funding although to a manageable extent. Doctors, clinicians, and support staff, on the other hand, remain staunch.

7.3 Clinical Protocol

Modified rotation advancement with small triangular flap and modified triangular flap repair for lip and Bardach, Furlow's, and Langenbeck for palate repair (depending upon the case) are the preferred surgical techniques which are employed at the center.

On an average, a patient needs to be admitted for 3–4 days in case of primary surgeries and suture removal in a lip surgery is typically done after 5 days but since pandemic absorbable sutures are being used for lip surgeries.

Moreover, the center has a well-structured follow-up system in place. Patients are contacted via phone 10 days post-surgery to check on their progress. Subsequent appointments take place in person at the hospital, through telemedicine center consultations or via an app-based telemedicine interface after 45 days, 6 months, and a year later. This follow-up regimen ensures that patients receive continued care and support.

Apart from the surgical procedures, the center also offers a variety of support services for the patients. These include nutrition and feeding counseling and support, oral health support, speech assessment and therapy, audiology, orthodontic treatment, and orthognathic treatment.

In addition to this, patient and attender accommodations, transport allowance, food services, and rehabilitation services are also available to aid patients in the journey of their recovery.

7.4 Community Outreach

The center's area of reach extends across the regions of Uttar Pradesh, Bihar, Jharkhand, and West Bengal. Some of the ways in which the center has reached needy patients include referrals from primary health care centers, cleft camps, center popularity (word of mouth) and through social media. In line with the center's commitment to community-based services, it has a tie-up with RBSK, which enables it to align its efforts with government initiatives and extend the reach to a larger number of patients in need.

7.5 Academic and Research Activities

Over the years, the center has been committed to training and mentoring plastic surgery and maxillofacial trainees significantly contributing to their professional development. Over 30 fellows have received training at the center for 2–4 weeks during their postgraduation and super specialization. The center has also been successful in providing training to more than 12 plastic surgeons and 3 maxillofacial surgeons. Notably, Smile Train has recently started comprehensive cleft fellowship at the center. Two seats are available for the same. There is a 1-year fellowship for plastic surgeons and maxillofacial surgeons and a 6 months certificate course for plastic surgeons. One maxillofacial surgeon is undergoing training in the current session.

The center is also involved in cleft genetic research since 2005 and has many original research papers in high impact journals to its name.

While the center has not developed specific patents or new techniques, its contributions to cleft care are indeed noteworthy. GS Memorial Plastic Surgery Hospital is the pioneer in cleft genetics in India. The center's efforts extend far beyond the laboratory and clinical settings. It has played a pivotal role in spreading awareness for the cause of cleft and several documentaries have been made highlighting the center's work. Among these documentaries, "Smile Pinki" stands out as a noteworthy achievement, having won the prestigious Academy Award (Oscar) in 2009 (2008 Academy Awards). This recognition propelled the documentary to international fame, making it one of the most widely viewed medical documentaries worldwide. The success of "Smile Pinki" brought about unprecedented attention to the issue of clefts.

7.6 Future Direction

The center's long-term vision includes a plan to build a larger, cutting-edge cleft, and craniofacial center that pushes the boundaries of excellence. The center envisions a state-of-the-art facility that not only provides comprehensive care but also promotes an environment of continuous learning and improvement. The center's message to the next generation of cleft care personnel is simple and clear: the impact of cleft surgery on a patient's life necessitates an in-depth knowledge of the underlying concepts. So, cleft care personnel should embrace this responsibility with utmost dedication keeping in mind that their work has the potential to transform lives. The center recommends future cleft centers to provide comprehensive treatment, all at one place. The center believes that there is a lack of comprehensive care, intense involvement, and engagement in the management of cleft patients. The field also lacks adequate focus on basic research and specialized craniofacial surgery. To bridge these gaps, healthcare professionals, researchers, policymakers, and the community must all come together to create a future wherein every individual with a cleft receives the best possible care and support.

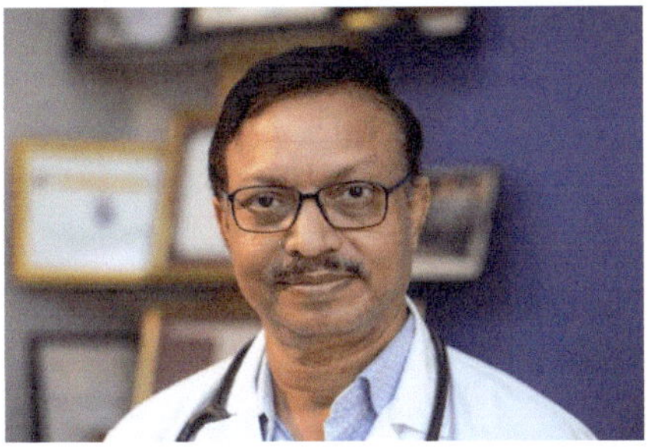

Dr. Subodh Singh (Plastic surgeon)

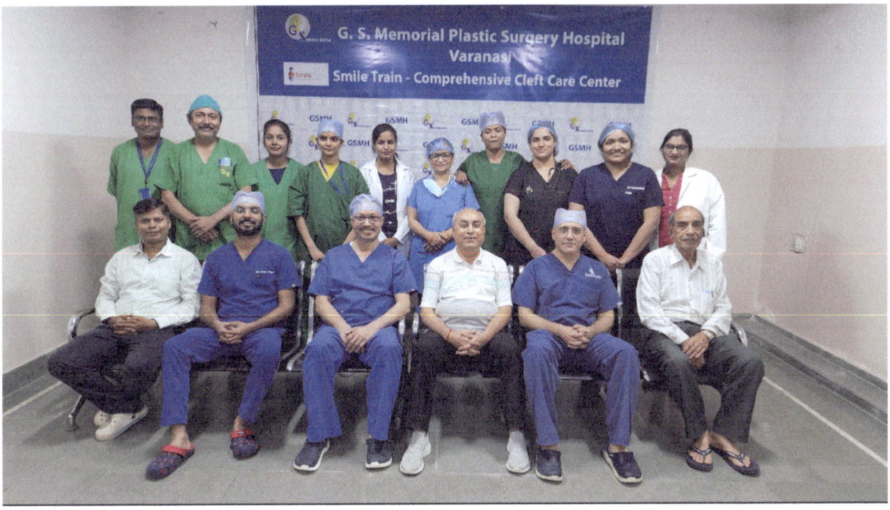

Sitting from left to right: **1. Dr. Abhinav Raj Gupta (orthodontist), 2. Dr. Ishan Singh (craniomaxillofacial surgeon), 3. Dr. Subodh Kumar Singh (Plastic Surgeon and Director of the Hospital), 4. Dr. K C Gupta (HoD Anaesthesiology), 5. Dr. Gaurav Nayyar (Plastic Surgeon), 6. Dr. SK Saigal (physician).** *Standing from left to right*: **1. Mr. Rewati Raman (senior Nursing Staff), 2. Dr. M K Tripathi (clinical coordinator), 3. Mrs. Dimple Maurya (Staff Nurse), 4. Ms. Neelam Yadav (Staff nurse), 5. Ms. Apurva Singh—nutritionist, 6. Mrs. Neeta Gupta (scrub nurse), 7. Ms. Shobha Kumari (critical care), 8. Dr. Pratima Rathor (paediateic anaesthesiologist), 9. Dr. Suprathima Sarita (maxillofacial surgeon—fellow in training), 10. Mrs. Sapna Mishra (speech language pathologist)**

Part III
The Central India Experience

Chapter 8
CARE CHL Hospital, Indore, Madhya Pradesh

Panchali Batra, Jaideep Singh Chauhan, Sarwpriya Sharma, Virag Bhatia, Simran Sharma, and Jagrati Junwal

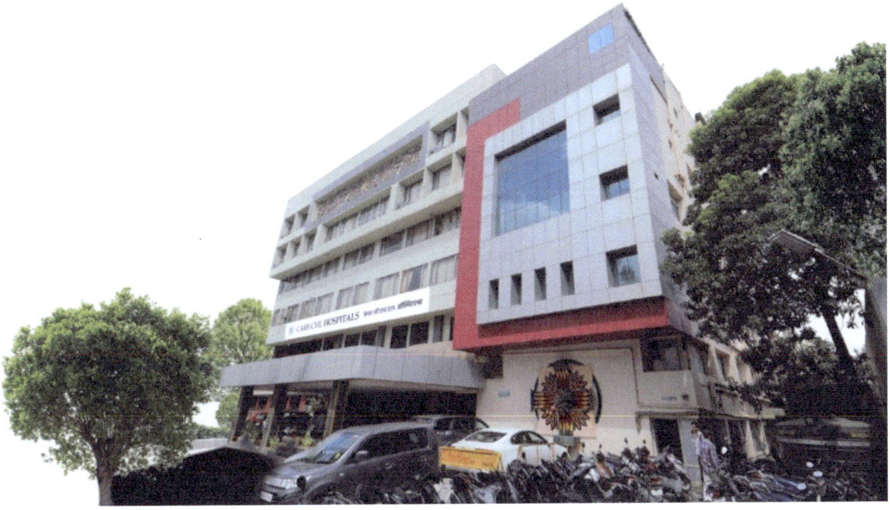

8.1 History and Milestones

Established on the 1st of December 2006 by Dr. Jaideep Singh Chauhan (Surgeon and Project Director, Smile Train) and funded by Smile Train, CARE CHL hospital has made a mark in cleft care and has achieved remarkable milestones. In 2008, this center collaborated with Smile Train and launched the Smile Train Van aimed to

P. Batra (✉)
Department of Orthodontics, Faculty of Dentistry, Jamia Millia Islamia, New Delhi, India
e-mail: p.batra@jmi.ac.in

J. S. Chauhan · S. Sharma · V. Bhatia · S. Sharma · J. Junwal
Smile Train Cleft Centre, CARE CHL Hospitals, Indore, India

P. Batra et al. (eds.), *The Cleft Care Framework in India*,
https://doi.org/10.1007/978-981-99-8968-3_8

reach remote locations so that cleft treatment is accessible to otherwise deprived population. The center went on to complete 5000 cleft surgeries and started a dedicated speech therapy unit for cleft patients in the year 2015. Orthodontic treatment for cleft patients started at the center in 2017 while nutritional program started in 2022. Smile Train owes much of its impressive growth and achievements to Dr. Jaideep Singh Chauhan. His extraordinary surgical skills combined with his leadership skills meant that he succeeded brilliantly in establishing one of its most successful centers globally. Equally significant contributions have come from Dr. Sarwpriya Sharma (Surgeon) and Ms. Jagrati Junwal (Speech pathologist) who demonstrated unwavering dedication toward promoting quality healthcare for cleft patients at Smile Train.

8.2 Present Scenario of the Center

CARE CHL Hospital is headed by Dr. Jaideep Singh. Along with Dr. Chauhan, the center has a great team of doctors, surgeons, clinicians, and support staff dedicated to providing exceptional care to the patients. This team includes Dr. Sarwpriya Sharma, a surgeon, Ms. Jagrati Junwal, a speech pathologist, and Dr. Virag Bhatia, an orthodontist. Since its inception, the center has been successful in operating 9700 cases till date. Surgical services, namely, lip surgery, palate surgery, and alveolar bone grafting and fistula closure surgeries are being offered by the center since 2006, cleft rhinoplasty started in 2007, orthognathic surgery and distraction osteogenesis in 2008 each and palate lengthening and VPI correction started in 2016. The center also provides rehabilitation services such as general dentistry, which has been into place since 2006, speech therapy and audiometry since 2015, orthodontics and nasoalveolar molding since 2017, nutritionist from 2022 and counselor from 2023. Diagnostic services being offered include dental radiography, computed tomography, and 2D Echocardiography since 2006 each, while nasoendoscopy and videofluroscopy are being offered since 2020.

8.3 Workflow

The center follows a defined work flow system which begins with OPD consultations followed by the admission of the patients in the hospital. Cleft surgery is performed the next day and the patients are discharged after 24–48 hours of surgery. Follow-up appointments are scheduled 2–4 weeks thereafter.

8.4 Clinical Protocol

The preferred surgical techniques employed for lip surgery at the center is Modified Millard, while Bardach is preferred for palate correction.

A patient needs to be admitted in the center for approximately 3 days in cases of primary surgeries and since resorbable sutures are being used, a patient does not need to report again just for suture removal. The follow-up time ranges from 2 weeks post-lip surgeries to 4 weeks post-palate surgeries for evaluation of the treatment outcome. Apart from all these services, there is a provision of accommodation for the patients/ attendants, free food for patients/ attendants as well as transportation allowance.

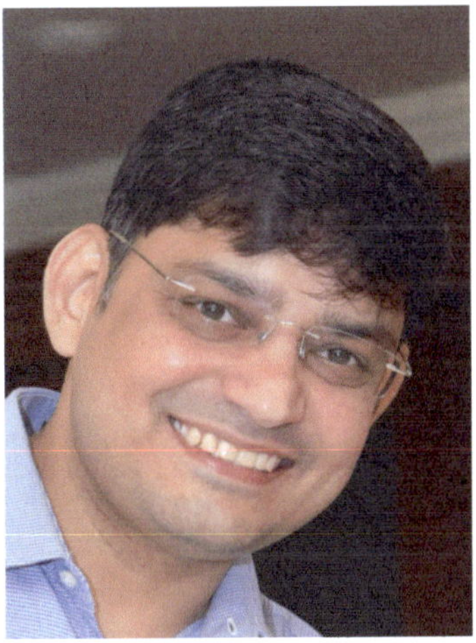

Dr. Jaideep Singh (Maxillofacial surgeon and project Director, Smile Train)

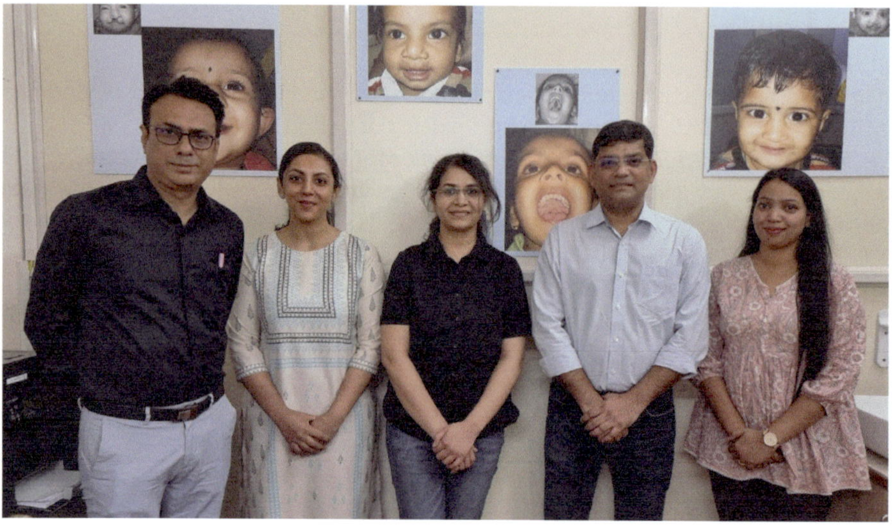

Cleft Care Team. (*From Right to Left:* **1. Ms. Jagrati Junwal – Speech Language Pathologist, 2. Dr. Jaideep Singh Chauhan – Surgeon and Project Director, Smile Train, 3. Dr. Sarwpriya Sharma – Surgeon, 4. Dr. Shreyasi Tiwari – Cleft Orthodontist, 5. Dr. Virag Bhatia – Cleft Orthodontist**)

Chapter 9
Sharad Pawar Dental College and Hospital, Acharya Vinobha Bhave Rural Hospital, Wardha, Maharashtra

Badri Thiruvenkatachari, Ranjit H. Kamble, Nitin Bhola, and Vikrant Jadhav

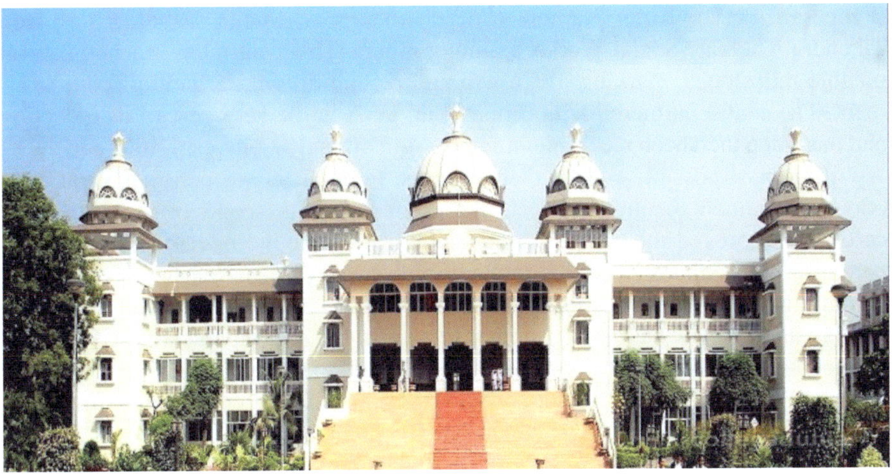

B. Thiruvenkatachari (✉)
Research, Sree Balaji Dental College and Hospital, BIHER, Chennai, India

Orthodontics, University of Manchester, Manchester, UK

R. H. Kamble
Smile Train Cleft Centre, Sharad Pawar Dental College & Hospital, Wardha, India

N. Bhola
Department of Oral & Maxillofacial Surgery, Sharad Pawar Dental College & Hospital, Wardha, India

V. Jadhav
Department of Orthodontics, Sharad Pawar Dental College & Hospital, Wardha, India

P. Batra et al. (eds.), *The Cleft Care Framework in India*,
https://doi.org/10.1007/978-981-99-8968-3_9

9.1 History

Sharad Pawar Dental College and Hospital, Acharya Vinobha Bhave Rural Hospital, located in Sawangi, Wardha Maharashtra has evolved as a renowned centre for cleft care in central India. Since its inception in 2007, the centre has made considerable progress in offering comprehensive cleft care services, conducting research, and teaching future cleft care specialists. Over the years, it has reached significant milestones, thanks to the leadership of its founder, Dr. Rajiv Borle (Oral Surgeon), the backing of Smile Train USA, its principal funding agency and the tireless efforts of its succeeding doctors and staff especially Dr. Nitin Bhola (Oral and Maxillofacial Surgeon and the Programme Director Smile train), Dr. Ranjit Kamble (Orthodontic treatment coordinator smile train), Dr. Pallavi Daigavane (Orthodontist), Dr. Suhas Jajoo (Plastic Surgeon), Dr. Shweta Pisulkar (Prosthodontist), Dr. Nilima Thosar (Pedodontist), Dr. Kiran Kamble (Speech therapist), Sunita Ganjudde (Nurse), Tikendra Khelkar (Social Worker), among others. This centre has reached several notable milestones, marking its growth and recognition in the field of cleft treatment. The centre partnered with Smile Train USA in the very year of its inception and has since then been receiving immense support and resources resulting in delivery of the best possible care to cleft patients. In 2017, it was certified as an orthodontic treatment centre which further broadened its scope of services. This certification proved the centre's proficiency in orthodontic interventions for cleft patients, foregrounding its commitment to integrated care approaches. The centre's recognition in 2019 as a national collaborator for Cleft Care India study by Jamia Millia Islamia, New Delhi was another feather in the cap which exhibited the centre's contribution in research besides its dedication to extensive knowledge in cleft treatment. In 2022, this centre was validated as a national collaborator for multicentric research in cleft NAMUC with BIHU Chennai too.

9.2 Present Scenario

This centre has been offering a wide range of surgical, rehabilitation as well as diagnostic services since the year 2007. The surgical services being offered include lip and palate surgeries, alveolar bone grafting, fistula closure, palate lengthening, orthognathic surgery, cleft rhinoplasty, and distraction osteogenesis while rehabilitation services include speech therapy, audiometry, orthodontics, nasoalveolar moulding, general dentistry, nutritionist, psychologist, counsellor, and ENT services (Grommet). In addition to these, the centre also offers advanced diagnostic services and is equipped with the latest technology in dental radiography, computed tomography, 2D echocardiography, and nasoendoscopy. The centre as a whole is committed to holistic care and support to cleft patients aiming to improve the patients' well-being manifolds.

Workflow System The centre has an organised workflow system which comprises of paediatric evaluation, PNAM (below 2 months), lip repair at 6–7 months of age, and palate repair at 15–17 months. Follow-up is scheduled for the evaluation of growth and development as well as to look for other issues, dental caries, for instance. Expansion procedures, if required are taken up at 7–8 years of age. If need arises, face masks are utilised for growth modulation. Fistula closure and ABG are taken up at 9–11 years of age followed by orthodontic procedures (with or without orthognathic surgeries). Revisions and rhinoplasty are carried out after the age of 18–19 years.

Challenges Faced by the Centre There are a few challenges that the centre faces. Instability of doctors and clinicians is one of them. A few trained clinicians have left the centre thereby requiring the recruitment and training of new clinicians. Instability of support staff, qualified speech language pathologist in particular is another challenge that the centre faces. Due to increase in the number of cleft care centres these days, the patient flow at this centre has also been affected in the last 2 years. Regardless of these challenges, the centre is committed to providing the best possible care to cleft patients.

Clinical Protocol The centre employs Millard rotation advancement flap for cleft lip while Bardach's Two Flap palatoplasty is the preferred surgical technique for cleft palate. The average duration of a patient's stay at the centre for primary surgeries is 2 days. This allows close monitoring of the patient's postoperative recovery. To ensure adequate healing, suture removal in case of a lip surgery is typically scheduled 7 days post the surgery. The centre ensures that there are regular telephonic conversations with the patients or their families to monitor progress, provide assistance to the patients or to address concerns if any. Furthermore, patients are provided with appointment cards which are a physical reminder of their follow-up appointments thereby reducing the chances of missing regular follow-ups. Apart from these, transport facility is being provided by the centre for the patients and accommodating parents so that lack of transportation does not hinder patients from receiving necessary interventions and care.

Community Outreach This centre has been treating patients from Vidharbha, Andhra Pradesh, as well as some parts of Madhya Pradesh and Chhattisgarh. There are various ways through which the centre reaches the needy, referrals from primary health care centres being one of them. Monthly cleft camps are conducted which further increase the centre's accessibility to the community. Positive feedbacks and word of mouth has led to the centre gaining popularity hence covering a greater audience in need of cleft care. The centre welcomes collaborations with government agencies, primary health centres, etc. with open arms which help in reaching out to more and more patients seeking cleft treatments and ensures that those in need get quality care and are treated successfully.

Academic and Research Activities The University is running "Fellowship in Cleft Orthodontics" wherein eight faculties have completed their fellowships from the year 2012 to 2022 whose names are enlisted herewith. Dr. Pallavi Daigavane completed her fellowship in 2012, followed by Dr. Priyank Niranjane in 2013, Dr. Rizwan Gilani in 2015, Dr. Garima Arya in 2017, Dr. R.H. Kamble in 2018, Dr. Jimmy Sangtani in 2020, Dr. Vikrant Jadhav in 2021, and Dr. Pratiksha Lakhe in 2022.

Certificate course were also conducted during 2012–2013. A total of 12 candidates were enrolled out of which six were internal and six externals. Dr. Puneet Batra was the adjunct faculty while Dr. P.V. Hazarey, Dr. Sunita Shrivastav, Dr. Ranjit Kamble, and Dr. Pallavi Daigavane were the coordinators for the same. Many scientific papers and research findings of the studies conducted at the centre have been published in both indexed and non-indexed journals. A new appliance used for the correction of shifted premaxilla called the PD Appliance has also been invented at the centre. Patent has been received for the same. The centre also reserves a copyright for a new classification system for UCLP infants to be treated with PSIO.

9.3 Future Direction

The centre envisions excellence in cleft care in central India with emphasis on evidence-based treatment modalities for cleft patients.

The centre's message to the next generation of cleft care personnel is that of encouragement and inspiration. Treating an individual having cleft deformity and restoring the facial and aesthetics is very satisfying job. It gives immense feeling of academic and clinical acumen and capabilities. Cleft care clinicians play a vital role for restoring the smiles of these patients. Young budding orthodontics/ surgeon should definitely venture into this field. The role of comprehensive knowledge about the research and studies being conducted in this domain cannot be ignored and this can be made possible by active participation in workshops, conferences, and online meetings with stalwarts and experts of the field. Evidence-based research and treatment should be put into practice to ensure the highest possible level of patient care.

Some areas of cleft care require attention in India. There is a lack of awareness among primary health workers and centres which delays the treatment. Another aspect which is currently lacking is timely referral to a specialist which is crucial for optimum treatment outcome. Remote areas lack funding and facilities too. Finally, there is a need to educate the general population about the prevalence of cleft defects and the importance of seeking timely and adequate interventions for the same.

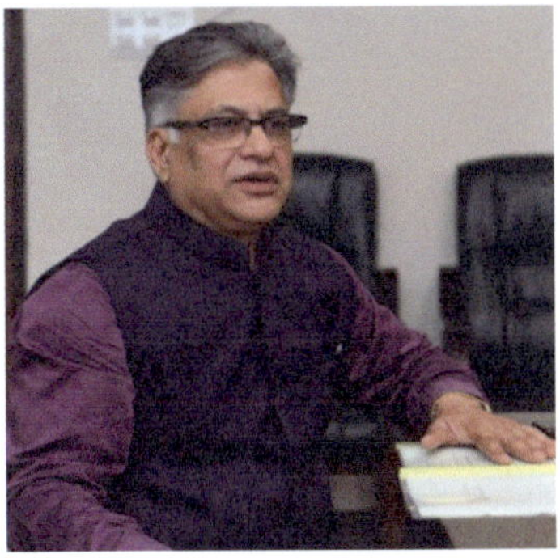

Dr. Rajiv Borle (Oral and Maxillofacial Surgeons)

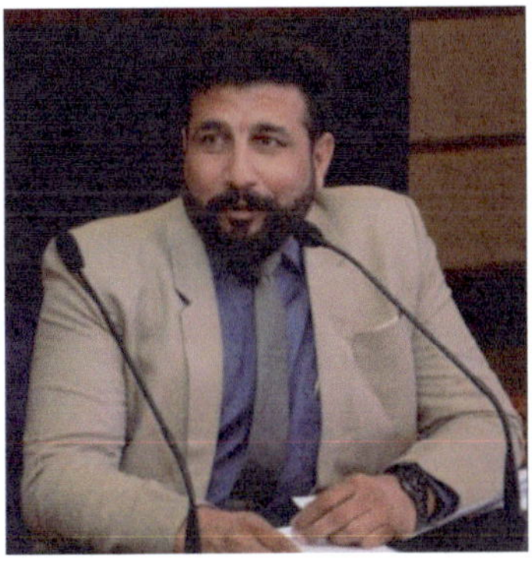

Dr. Nitin Bhola

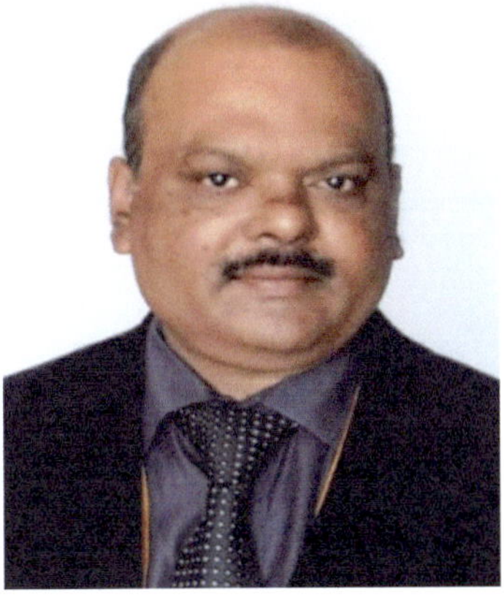

Dr. Ranjit Kamble (Orthodontist)

Part IV
The East India Experience

Chapter 10
Guwahati Comprehensive Cleft Care Centre (GC4), Guwahati, Assam

Deborah Sybil, Hiteswar Sarma, and Dipul Malakar

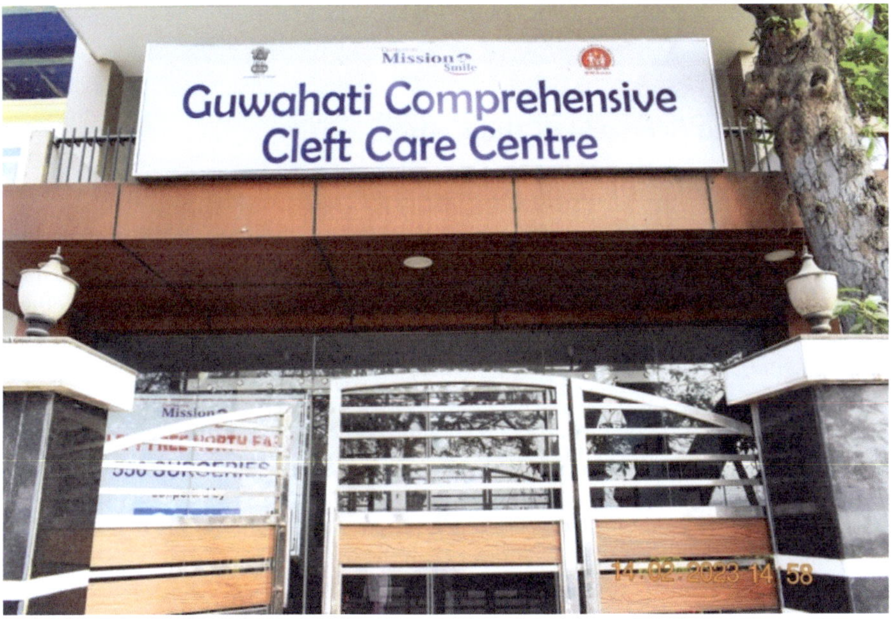

10.1 History of the Center

Established on 9th May 2011, Guwahati Comprehensive Cleft Care Centre (GC4), Mission smile is a center devoted to providing comprehensive care for cleft patients. GC4 has achieved some noteworthy milestones ever since it started. In a matter of

D. Sybil (✉)
Department of Oral Surgery, Faculty of Dentistry, Jamia Millia Islamia, New Delhi, India

H. Sarma · D. Malakar
Guwahati Comprehensive Cleft Care Center, Mission Smile, Kolkata, India

P. Batra et al. (eds.), *The Cleft Care Framework in India*,
https://doi.org/10.1007/978-981-99-8968-3_10

just 1 year, 5000 surgeries were successfully carried out at the center. This number increased to 10,000 in 2013 and 20,000 in the year 2019. Not only this, the center has also established collaborations with government bodies. The center entered MoU with Meghalaya Government for cleft care in 2012 and this was renewed again in 2014.

Ranjit Barthakur, the Chairman of Mission Smile, is the pioneer of GC4 and has been instrumental in taking the center forward over the years. His vision and restless efforts have helped create GC4 a premier cleft care center. Dr. Alex Campbell, USA, is another esteemed doctor who has contributed to the center's growth with his expertise and knowledge. National Health Mission, Assam and TATA TRUST help the center financially by providing funds to expand and continue its services.

10.2 Present Scenario of the Center

The center is headed by Conrad Dennis. The center has a dedicated team of Surgeons, anesthetists, pediatrician, dentists, nurses, speech therapist, and support staff without whose unwavering support the success of this center would not have been possible. The medical team consists of Dr. Hiteswar Sarma (Surgeon, Medical Director), Dr. Kamal Kayal (Staff Anesthetist), Dr. Suryya Kumar Debnath (Pediatrician), Dr. Gyanshree Khound (Anesthetist), Dr. Sweta Parna Deb (Trainee Surgeon), Dr. Anandita Paul (Dentist), Dr. Pranjal Bora (Anesthetist on call), Dr. Hemanta Kalita (Surgeon on call), and Dr. Dipjyoti Baruah (Orthodontist). The support team and staff include Dipul Malakar (Assistant GM- Program and Partnership), Jonashree Das (Senior Manager-Administration), Arem Chiru (Nursing Head), Manika Deka (Assistant Manager-Patient Care), Hridayananda Bhuyan (Executive-Accounts), Hemanta Sarma (Anesthesia Technician), Mubidur Rahman (Executive-Patient Recruitment), Aparna Dahal (Speech Therapist), Moromi Nath (Sr. Executive-Nutrition Program), Ajoy Borah (Executive-Patient Imaging), Manash Baruah (Executive-Patient Care), Hare Krishna Sharma (Executive-Patient Care), Arabolin Kharkongor (Staff Nurse), Amy Grace Moore Mihsill (Staff Nurse), Kaikho Chiipfohra (NHM Staff Nurse), Onima Marak (NHM Staff Nurse), Seiminlim Chongloi (NHM Staff Nurse), Moni Deori Gogoi (NHM Staff Nurse), Tarali Tahbildar (NHM Staff Nurse), Jinti Das (NHM Staff Nurse), Bandana Buragohain (NHM Staff Nurse), Nandini Sinha (NHM Staff Nurse), Pinkumoni Deka (NHM Staff Nurse), Rizwana Kharbithai (NHM Staff Nurse), Juri Deka (NHM Staff Nurse), Namita Sarma (NHM Staff Nurse), Manglianching Kamei (NHM Staff Nurse).

The center has operated a total of 22,538 cases till January 2023. GC4 provides a range of surgical services, namely, lip surgery, palate surgery, alveolar bone grafting, fistula closure, palate lengthening, VPI correction, and cleft rhinoplasty. The center also provides rehabilitation services which include speech therapy, audiometry, orthodontics, nasoalveolar molding, general dentistry, nutritionist, psychologist, counselor, and ENT services (Grommet) besides dental radiography for diagnostic purposes.

10.3 Workflow

It involves several well organized stages and begins with pre-screening of patients in district/other state followed by screening comprising of registration, multiple physical examinations done by nurse, pediatrician, surgeon, anesthesiologist, dentist, and Speech Therapist. This is followed by PIT, Lab Test, and Final Station (Clinical Coordinator). The admission process begins with giving the screening update to the patients and guardian and the surgery is scheduled. The patient is then admitted to pre-operative ward. The day of the surgery commences with pre-operative visit by the medical team in the ward followed by child life counseling and then the patient is taken to the operation theater for surgery. The patient is then transferred to the recovery room and post-operative ward. The patient is discharged the next morning with post-operative check-up instructions. The first post-operative follow-up is scheduled after 7 days, while the second and third follow-ups are scheduled in 2 and 6 months, respectively.

The center receives funding from various sources. The principal funding agencies are the National Health Mission Assam, Meghalaya, and Tripura. Smile Asia, Singapore also provides funding. In addition to these, the center also receives support from other donors such as Colgate, Bajaj, OIL, ONGC, IOCL, and others.

The center faces a few challenges which need addressal for continued provision of quality care. Inadequate funding and instability of doctors and clinicians and support staff pose barriers to the center's growth. Patient flow is another factor which needs management. The center has also experienced infrastructural problems after being relocated from its original facility to an adjoining new location temporarily in 2022, as per the government notification.

10.4 Clinical Protocol

The surgical techniques at the center are chosen based on the type of clefts. For unilateral (incomplete) cleft lip Fisher's technique, for unilateral (complete) cleft lip, Modified Mohler's technique and for bilateral cleft lip (incomplete and complete) Millard's technique is used at the center, while for incomplete (unilateral and bilateral) cleft palate Langenback's technique and for complete (unilateral and Bilateral) cleft palate Bardach's technique is preferred. For primary surgeries, the average duration of stay of the patient in the hospital is 2 days. The patient does not need to return to the center for suture removal as resorbable sutures are used at GC4.

The center has a well-organized follow-up system in place to evaluate patients development after surgery. The first post-operative appointment is set for 7 days after the surgery. The second follow-up is scheduled 2 months later, and the third is conducted in the sixth month. Various support services are provided at the center for the comfort and convenience of the patients and their attendants. Free accommodation and food are provided to the patients and the attendants during their stay at the hospital. The center also provides to and fro transportation to patient and attendants. Smile bags containing toothpaste, toothbrush, soap, mirror, comb, towel and food bags containing milk, bread, and juice are also offered by the center.

10.5 Community Outreach

The area of reach of the center is MMC Hospital, Panbazar, Guwahati-1. The center has reached to the needy patients through referrals from primary health care centers, cleft camps, and center popularity (word of mouth).

Some community-based services that this center offers/supports include community health workers awareness on cleft care services at district level, BLS/ACLS/ nursing training and education, pre-screening camps at the district level, district outreach medical camps for postoperative patients, surgery outreach camp, and students internship/training/volunteering.

10.6 Academic and Research Activities

The center has successfully conducted fellowship which is cleft surgery training program (CSTP) wherein 16 fellows from India and abroad were given trainings. Some of these fellows are now working successfully across the country and the globe.

The center has also been actively engaged in several funded projects, particularly in multicentric cleft studies supported by ICMR and a total of about 24–25 scientific papers have been published in different journals.

One of the notable contributions by the center in cleft care is the development of a modified technique for unilateral complete lip repair, known as the GC4 modified Mohler's technique.

10.7 Future Direction

The center plans and strives to develop as a research and training hub for Cleft Care in India and South -East Asia and believes that cleft care must be developed as a distinguished branch of health care (Community health care).

The center recommends that every cleft care center should strive to be a comprehensive unit, incorporating not just medical and surgical interventions but also cleft nutrition.

One of the primary areas where cleft care in India falls short is in its comprehensive approach and by addressing this gap, the overall quality of care provided to cleft patients can increase manifolds.

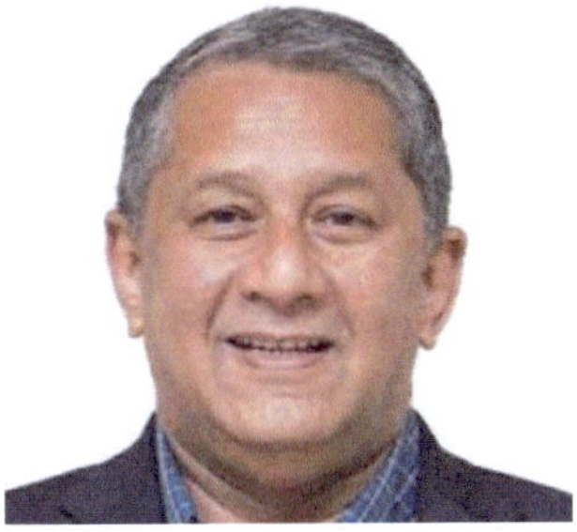

Dr. Ranjit Barthakur (Founder)

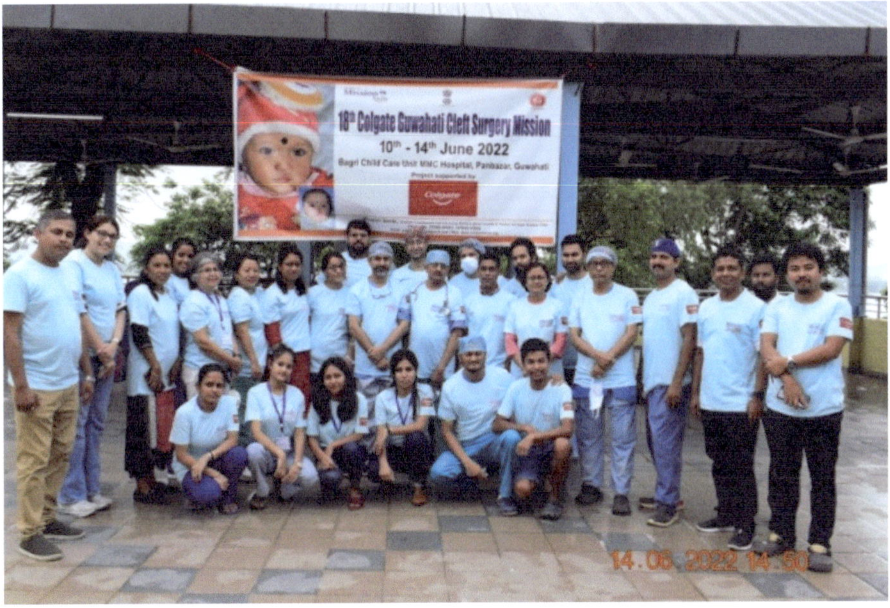

Mission Smile Team

Chapter 11
IGIMS Comprehensive Cleft Care, Patna, Bihar

Panchali Batra and Priyankar Singh

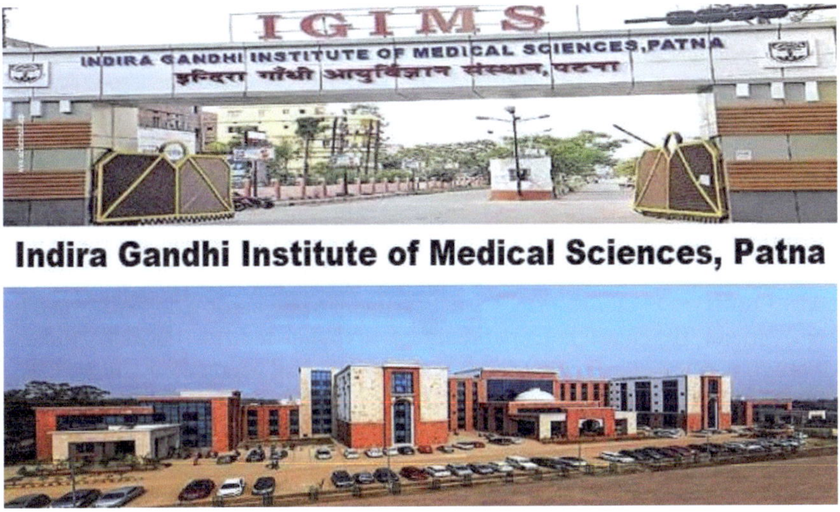

History of the Center Indira Gandhi Institute of Medical Sciences Comprehensive Cleft Care, Patna started in December 2019 by Dr. Priyankar Singh with the invaluable support of Prof. Dr. N.R. Biswas, then Director IGIMS, Patna. The center achieved phenomenal milestones within a short time span of just around 2.5 years. The center embarked upon its journey with its first case of CLCP, in the year 2019 by Dr. Priyankar Singh. Subsequently, the center got RBSK funding support from RBSK (Rashtriya Bal Swasthya Karyakram), Govt. of Bihar and was recognized as the first government funded cleft center in Bihar as an autonomous government tertiary institute in 2020. Almost 100 cases were successfully operated upon under

P. Batra (✉)
Department of Orthodontics, Faculty of Dentistry, Jamia Millia Islamia, New Delhi, India
e-mail: p.batra@jmi.ac.in

P. Singh
Indira Gandhi Institute of Medical Sciences, Patna, India

P. Batra et al. (eds.), *The Cleft Care Framework in India*,
https://doi.org/10.1007/978-981-99-8968-3_11

Dr. Singh's supervision even in the COVID-19 era. The center finally got a dedicated Cleft OT and six bedded ward especially for comprehensive cleft care in 2022. The present director IGIMS, (Prof.) Dr. Bindey Kumar who himself is a stalwart pediatric surgeon has been like wind beneath the wings of this comprehensive cleft center to take it up to new heights. The medical superintendent, (Prof.) Dr. Manish Mandal has immensely helped in providing his wholehearted support for procurement of the required infrastructure and instruments for the betterment of cleft center here at IGIMS, PATNA. The Chief PGIDER is Prof. (Dr.) A. K. Sharma under whose guidance the Cranio-Maxillo-Facial unit has created milestones.

Present Scenario of the Center The center comprises a team of skilled doctors, surgeons, clinicians, and support staff. Dr. Priyankar Singh, the pioneer and a dedicated and experienced cleft surgeon himself, serves as the center head cleft center incharge (Prof.) Dr. Aman Kumar, the Nodal Officer for RBSK, is a strong pillar in helping such needy patients to avail free treatment and has turned no stone unturned to take team RBSK at IGIMS across the rubicon. Prominent faculties and the Head of the Department of Anesthesia Prof. (Dr.) P. K. Dubey and the head of trauma and emergency Dr. Raj Bahadur Singh has always been supportive and are on toes to handle any emergency peri-operatively. The Department of Pediatric Medicine headed by Prof.(Dr.) Jayant Kumar, The Department of Pediatric Surgery headed by Prof.(Dr.) Vineet Thakur, The Department of ENT headed by Prof.(Dr.) Rakesh Kumar Singh is an asset for the comprehensive care for all needy cleft children. The Department of Psychiatry headed by Prof.(Dr.) Rajesh Kumar has been of immense help in psychological establishment in the society for such children. Several OT Technicians and Ward Nurses are some of the noted members of the team who work 24*7 to take care of such kids in designated ward and operating room. Nearly, 800 patients are registered at the center with 500 having successfully received surgical interventions even though restrictions were imposed by the COVID-19 pandemic in 2020 thereby leading to a significant reduction in the number of surgeries performed. The center boasts of providing state-of-the-art surgical, rehabilitation, and diagnostic procedures. It specializes in lip and palate surgeries, alveolar bone grafting, fistula closure, palate lengthening, VPI correction, orthognathic surgery, Cleft rhinoplasty, and distraction osteogenesis. Various rehabilitation services which are being provided here include speech therapy, audiometry, orthodontics, nasoalveolar molding, general dentistry, nutritionist, psychologist, counselor, and ENT services. The center also has a dedicated unit for diagnosis which includes dental radiography, computed tomography, 2D echocardiography, nasoendoscopy, and videofluroscopy.

Workflow system at the center: The workflow system at the center follows a strict protocol to ensure the safety and well-being of the patients. Patients come not just from Bihar but also from neighboring states and even Nepal to seek treatment at this center. A comprehensive preoperative assessment is performed which includes blood tests, chest X-rays, 2D echocardiography, pediatric check-ups, pre-anesthetic evaluations, and testing for COVID-19. While the number of surgeries performed may be lower than that of some private funded NGOs, the center prioritizes quality over quantity.

The center does face a few challenges in the form of inadequate funding, poverty, and a lack of cleft awareness among the general population. Despite these challenges the center strives to provide quality care to cleft patients.

11.1 Clinical Protocol

The preferred surgical technique at this center for lip and palate correction is Millard's rotation advancement flap. For primary surgeries, patients are normally admitted for 1 day before the surgery and 3 days after the completion of the surgery. The surgeons at the center generally use Vicryl sutures, which are absorbable and so do not need suture removal. 7-0 and 6-0 Vicryl sutures are put for lip surgeries. After discharge, the patients are scheduled for evaluation every seventh day. Patients are then followed up every 2 months for the first year. After that follow-up appointments are scheduled as and when required.

The center provides patient and attender accommodation, transport allowance, food services, rehabilitation services, surgery, and medication free of cost.

11.2 Community Outreach

IGIMS comprehensive cleft care is located at the center of Bihar and is therefore easily accessible to all. The center has implemented different ways to ensure that patients avail benefits from here. It receives referrals from primary health care workers and is associated with all Anganwadi and ASHA workers. Cleft camps are conducted every 2 months by RBSK officials which further expands the center's outreach. Since, it is the only government tertiary care in the region, this center has gained a great degree of popularity among the population by word of mouth.

11.3 Academic and Research Activities

Although the main fellowship program is awaiting Bihar government's approval, the center has started an observership program wherein two observers/fellows have already been trained at the center. Two of the noteworthy research projects carried out by the center includes Evaluating the effectiveness of NAM in complete unilateral non-syndromic CL/P children, multicentric with Dr. Badri as PI and Evaluating the transcriptional gene analysis in non-syndromic CL/P children being conducted at IGIMS by intra mural funds.

The center's most notable achievement in the last 2 years has been a marked reduction in the number of patients moving out of the state to seek treatment. They have started trusting IGIMS, Patna for complex surgeries too which speaks volumes about the center's dedication toward quality care. The center's active involvement in new research projects has yielded promising results in cleft genetics.

11.4 Future Direction

The center is on its path to becoming a state-of-the-art comprehensive cleft care center for the entire east India region, providing treatment at zero cost. The center focuses on combining the traditional "OLD is GOLD" surgical techniques with newer modifications and technologies, so that the patients receive the best possible treatment. While it is important to keep up with the latest researches and advancements in the field, it is equally important to recognize the importance of established practices and techniques. By integration of past knowledge and present breakthroughs, the quality of cleft treatment can further be stepped up. Rather than focusing on the number of surgeries performed, it is crucial to level up the treatment quality.

Cleft care in India faces various challenges, the lack of awareness among the general population being one of them. Another challenge that cleft centers often face is the lack of funds as well as infrastructure to continue unhindered services. A shortage of trained surgeons and clinicians specialized in cleft care is another issue which needs to be addressed. Moreover, many states lack government support making it difficult for cleft care centers to expand and provide treatment to those in need.

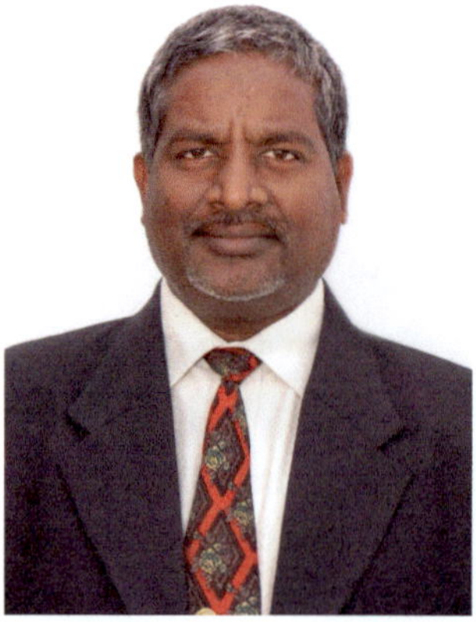

Prof.(Dr.) Bindey Kumar DIRECTOR, IGIMS, PATNA

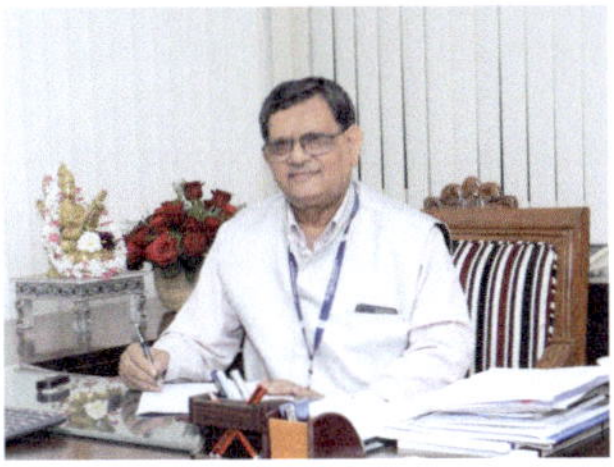

Prof.(Dr.) N.R.Biswas, Ex- DIRECTOR, IGIMS, PATNA

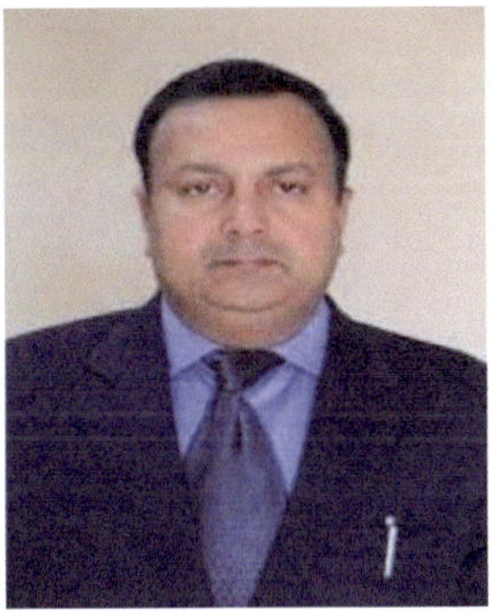

Prof.(Dr.) Manish Mandal (MEDICAL SUPRINTENDENT, IGIMS, PATNA)

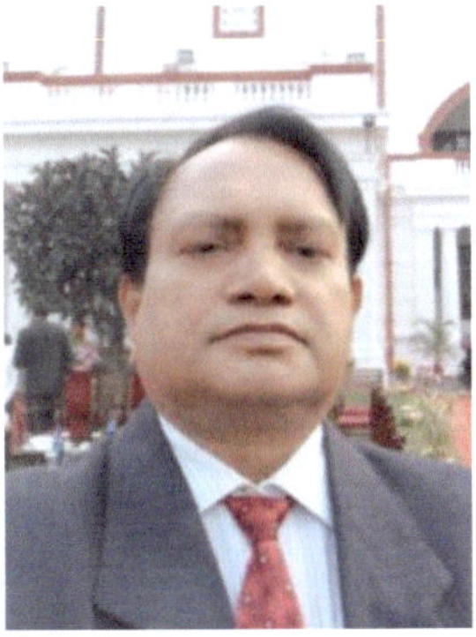

Prof.(Dr.) A.K.Sharma (CHIEF, PGIDER, IGIMS, PATNA)

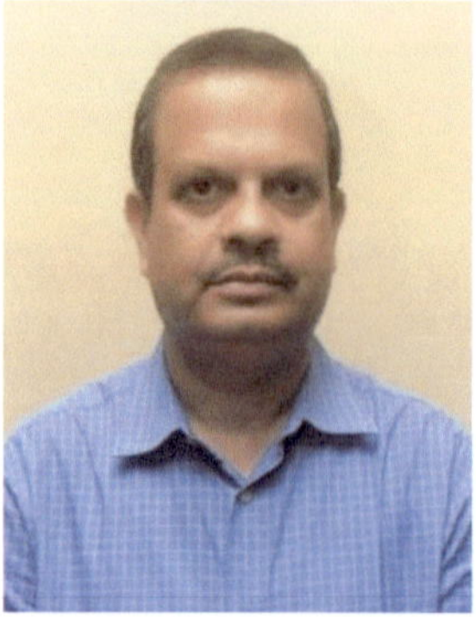

Prof.(Dr.) Aman Kumar (NODAL OFFICER, R.B.S.K, IGIMS, PATNA)

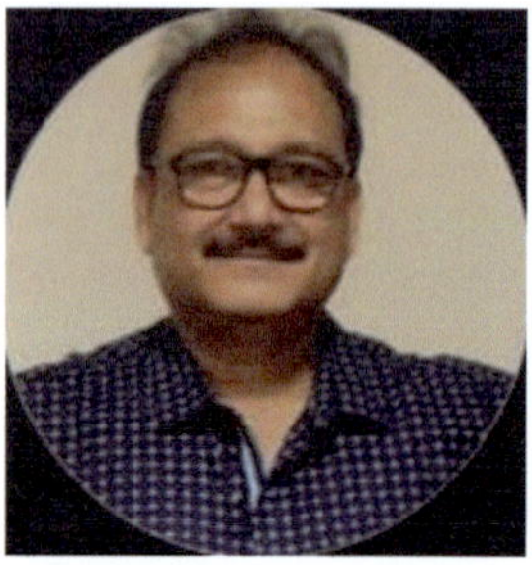

Prof.(Dr.) P.K.Dubey (Head of Anesthesia)

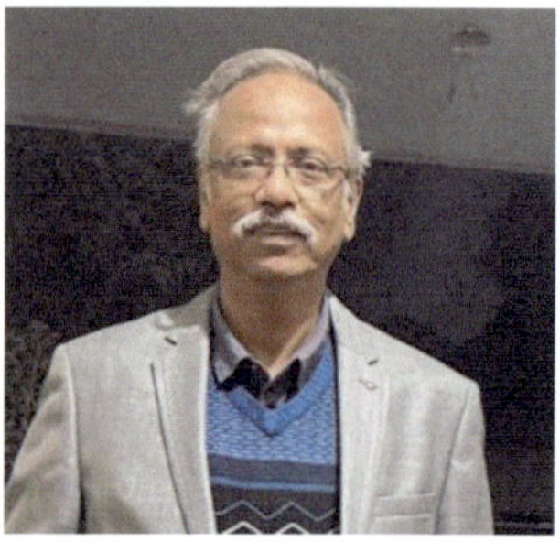

Prof.(Dr.) Jayant Kumar (Head of Pediatric Medicine)

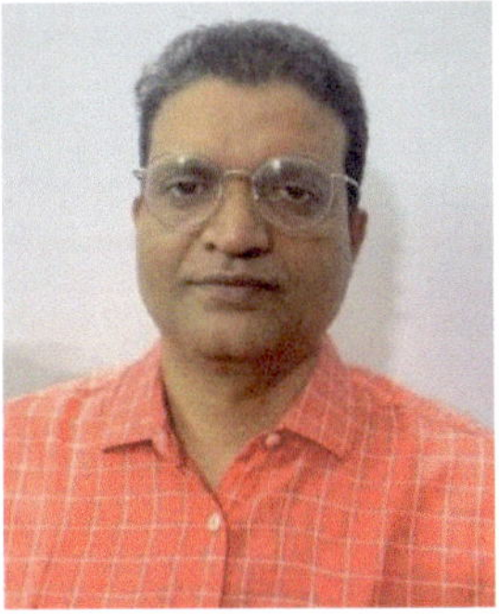

Prof.(Dr.) Vineet Thakur (Head of Pediatric Medicine)

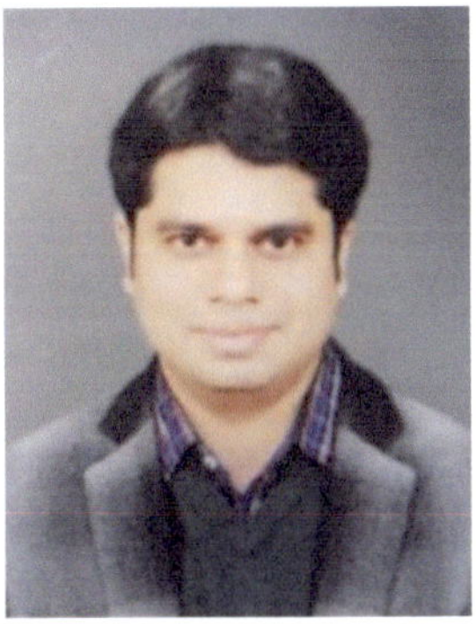

Dr. Raj Bhadur Singh (Head of Trauma & Emergency)

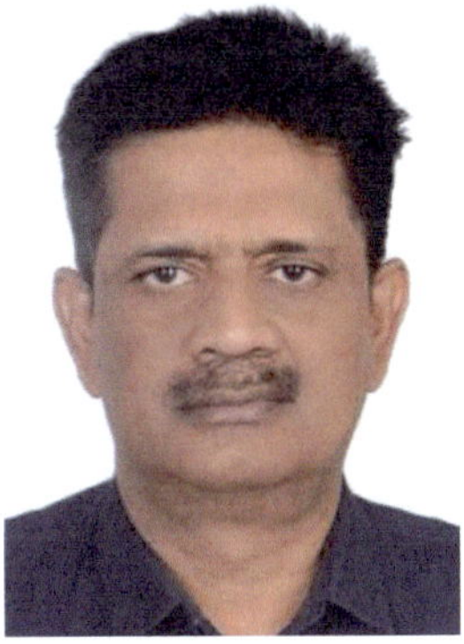

Prof. (Dr.) Rakesh Kumar Singh (HEAD, ENT)

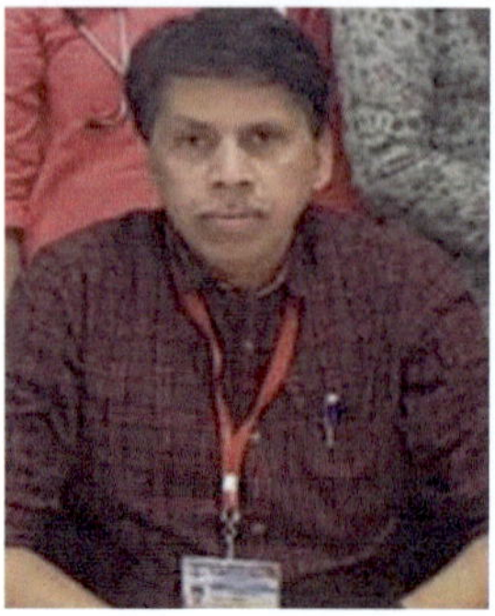

Prof. (Dr.) Rajesh Kumar (HEAD, PSYCHIATRY)

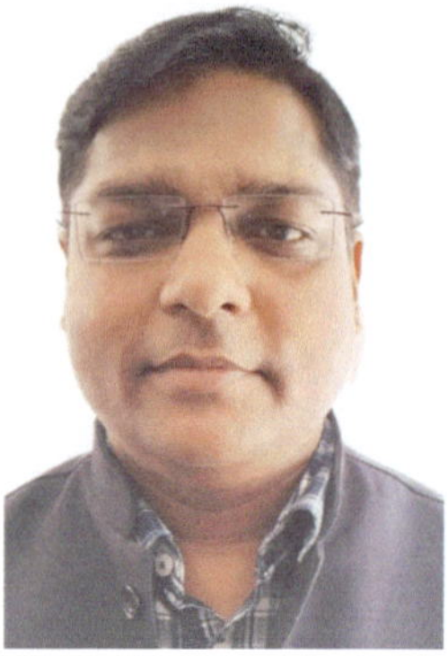

Dr. Priyankar Singh (Cleft surgeon and unit in charge)

Chapter 12
ABMSS Comprehensive Cleft Care (CCC) Centre, Kolkata, West Bengal

Badri Thiruvenkatachari, Dushyant Prasad and Siddhartha Chatterjee

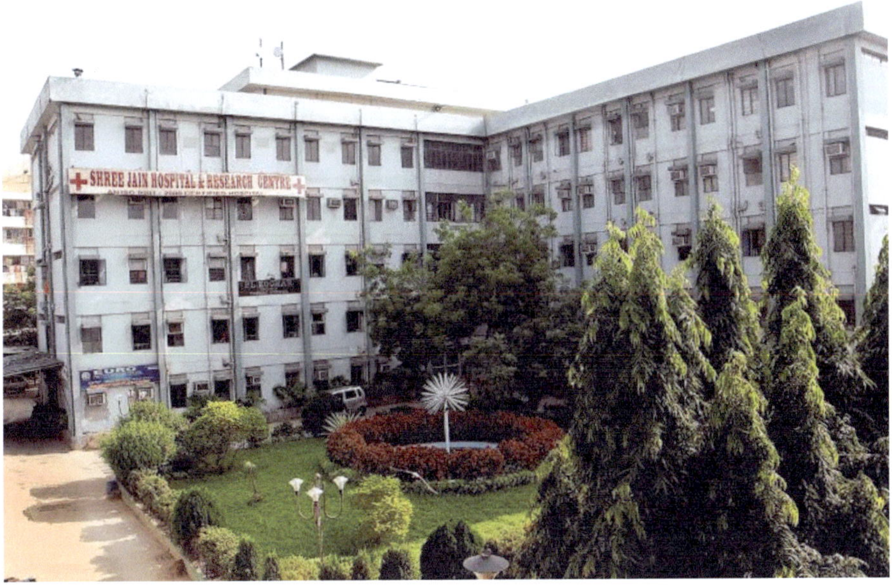

B. Thiruvenkatachari (✉)
Sree Balaji Dental College and Hospital, BIHER, Chennai, India

University of Manchester, Manchester, UK

D. Prasad · S. Chatterjee
Shree Jain Hospital Howrah, Kolkata, India
e-mail: dushyant.prasad@abmss.in

P. Batra et al. (eds.), *The Cleft Care Framework in India*,
https://doi.org/10.1007/978-981-99-8968-3_12

12.1 History

The ABMSS Comprehensive Cleft Care (CCC) Centre located at Shree Jain Hospital Kolkata is a pioneering medical centre in India's Eastern Region.

The centre, which opened in November 2017, began as a cleft care centre and eventually grew into a comprehensive cleft care centre in 2019. The hospital, situated in West Bengal's Howrah district, is well-known for its paediatric and gynaecology services. The CCC Centre at Shree Jain Hospital answers the region's need for comprehensive cleft care.

Under the able guidance of Dr. Siddhartha Chatterjee, the centre's director, the CCC team is committed to providing comprehensive care to those with cleft deformities. The team consists of skilled professionals, including Dr. Nidhi Bodra, a cleft fellow, as well as Dr. Sayantan Mukherjee, Dr. Balram Nishad, Dr. Rachana Chowdhury, Dr. Sourav Jash, Dr. Priyabrata Sit (Anaesthesiologist), Dr. Krishnendu (Orthodontist), Dr. Tuhina Ghosh (Pedodontist), Dr. Kalamuddin (Paediatrician), speech therapist Ms. Beauty Singh, and social worker Mr. Saharul Laskar. Together, they ensure the smooth working of the centre's services.

Since its beginning, the ABMSS Comprehensive Cleft Care Centre has treated a large number of patients. Despite the obstacles faced by the centre due to the pandemic in 2020, the centre successfully completed 1876 cleft surgeries and offered comprehensive treatment to a large number of children in West Bengal. These accomplishments demonstrate Dr. Chatterjee's continuous commitment to improving the lives of children born with clefts in the region.

The centre's primary funding agency is ABMSS which happens to be the second largest cleft NGO in the country.

12.2 Present Scenario

The centre provides all primary and secondary cleft surgeries including VPI Correction, ENT surgeries, orthognathic surgeries including distraction osteogenesis and the entire circle of care CCC services including NAM, Nutrition, Speech therapy, ENT (Surgeries too to prevent hearing loss), Dental, Orthodontics, Audiometry, and hearing aids. The centre not only provides primary surgeries but also offers secondary procedures including distraction osteogenesis as the child grows up, ensuring comprehensive care throughout their journey into adulthood.

This centre also provides a complete diagnostic infrastructure, which includes in-house 2D ECHO, CT scans, ultrasound scans, videolaryngoscopy, nasal endoscopy, and an entire range of blood examinations. The centre's ability to meet the complicated requirements of children with congenital disorders is further enhanced by this diverse set of resources.

12.3 Workflow

The centre's workflow involves outreach work across West Bengal and neighbouring states. An exclusive field animator conducts field work all through the year to identify patients in need. A good proportion of cases also do walk in through professional referral and word of mouth. Once the patients arrive at the centre, they undergo counselling for CCC based on the stage and diagnosis that they present with. They are then registered in to the database and are issued a Cleft Passport with unique number, following which they go through work up and CCC referral. Patients are regularly checked for their dental hygiene during their visit to centre.

The ABMSS Comprehensive Cleft Care Centre faces several challenges which include the fragile social work ecosystem including the logistical challenges in transportation for patient families, a lack of beds and wards for accompanying family members, difficulties with local administration's understanding of the centre's work in rural areas, ever increasing costs associated with recruiting patients and involving intermediaries, regular demand from hospital, and other team members to ensure pay parity, and limited resources for special investigations of syndromic children along with the challenges of following school children especially after their return to school following pandemic.

Despite these challenges, the ABMSS Comprehensive Cleft treatment Centre at Shree Jain Hospital remains committed to its purpose of providing comprehensive treatment to individuals with cleft lip and palate, allowing them to live fulfilling lives.

The centre mainly utilises Millard and Fischer technique for Cleft lip repair, Bardach's technique, and Traditional Vonlagenback's technique for incomplete cleft palate and a Furlows for Submucous cleft palate. The average stay for most patients is 2–3 days in the hospital with most of them coming back on Day 10 for a checkup along with suture removal.

12.4 Clinical Protocol

The centre's comprehensive cleft care programme offers an organised treatment plan for children from the time they are born until they have their primary lip surgery done. Initially, the child visits the centre every 10 days for nasoalveolar moulding. After the lip closure, bimonthly checkups are scheduled until the palate is repaired. Once the palate is repaired, the child has annual visits for speech evaluation and stimulation until therapy begins at the age of 3.5 years. These appointments also involve ENT and dental checkups. As the child grows, procedures such as speech improvement surgery, lip revision, or fistula repair may be required, which are done between the ages of 4 and 6 years old based on appropriate indications. Then the child begins mixed dentition orthodontics to expand the arch or initiate growth modifying therapy before bone grafting, which is usually done between 9 and 11 years of age based on the stage of canine eruption. Annual visits continue to monitor dental and ENT health, speech progress, and overall growth during this entire period. They undergo presurgical orthodontics thereafter and are ready for jaw advancement and final rhinoplasty following their adolescence growth cessation.

Almost all Surgical and CCC services are free along with transportation and food support for patient and family during each visit. To broaden their reach and raise awareness, the centre uses a camp van to conduct awareness camps and bring in patients from nearby areas.

12.5 Community Outreach

The centre covers not only half the state of West Bengal but also bordering districts of Bihar and Jharkhand. Patients come for treatment through field animator-organised camps, professional referrals, and word of mouth. The centre has collaborations with the Satya Sai Foundation and Rural Health Care Foundation to identify patients needing surgeries.

12.6 Academic and Research Activities

In addition to providing quality care, the centre also supports fellowship programmes since 2018. Currently, four fellows have completed the programme.

12.7 Future Direction

The centre hopes to promote visibility through electronic media, increase access to CCC services, and raise awareness in order to reach out to more people in need of cleft care. The long-term goal is to provide comprehensive cleft care for the entire region. The centre is a strong believer in the fact that surgical intervention alone is insufficient, and it pushes for government intervention and support for CCC, including parental aid for the provision of full scope treatment for children with cleft problems in the region.

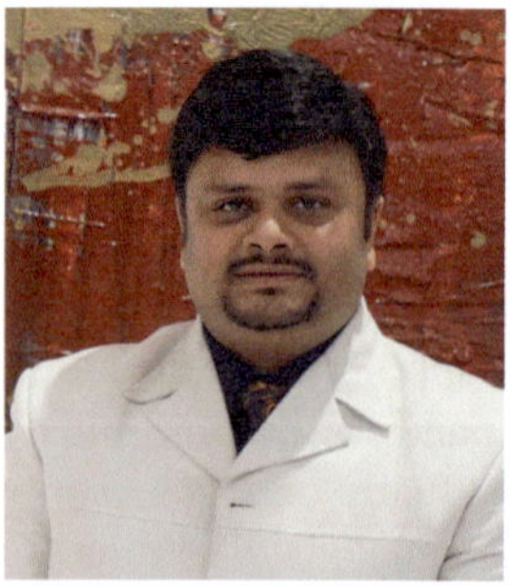

Dr. Siddhartha Chatterjee (Oral and Maxillofacial Surgeon)

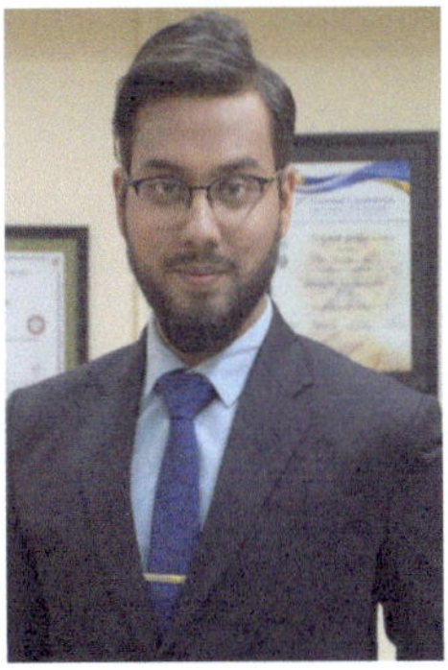

Dr. Krishnendu Chatterjee (Orthodontist)

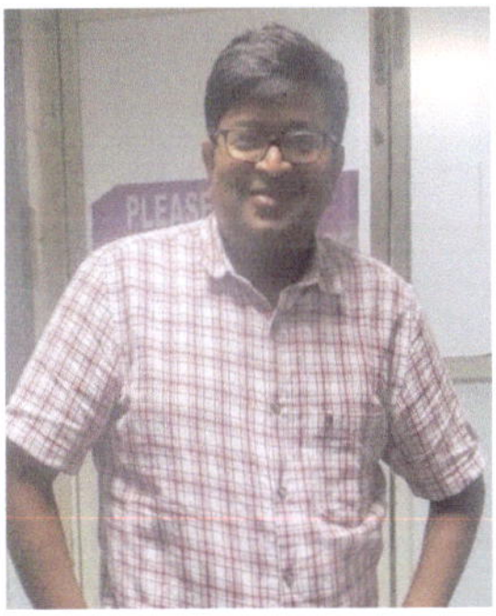

Dr. Balaram Nisad (Anaesthesiologist)

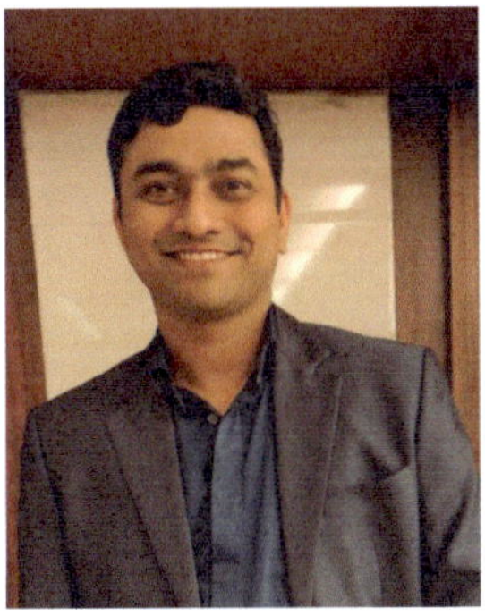

Dr. Sarah Jash (Anaesthesiologist)

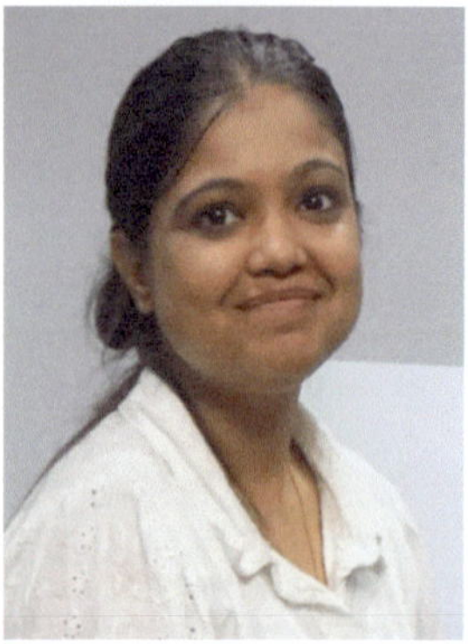

Dr. Beauty Singh (Speech therapist)

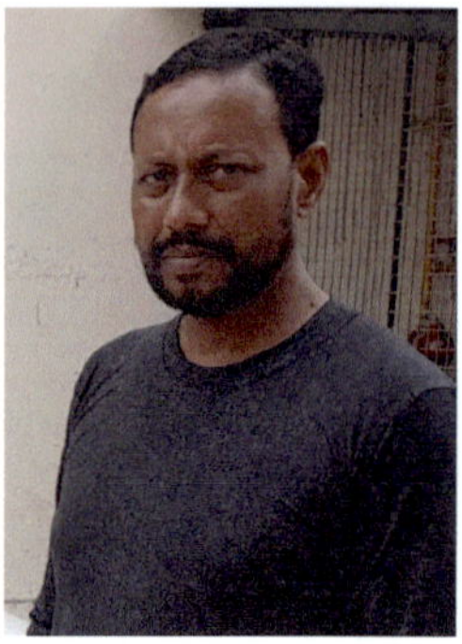

Dr. Saharul Laskar (Project Animator)

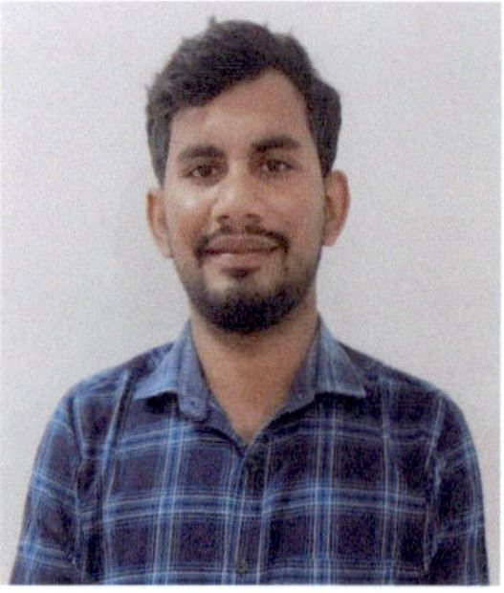

Prem Kumar Singh (Data entry operator)

Chapter 13
Ashwini Hospital, Cuttack, Orissa

Deborah Sybil, Subrat Kumar Jena, Shibani Das, Surya Kanta Das, Shubhasmita Mahakud, and Swaleha Shirin

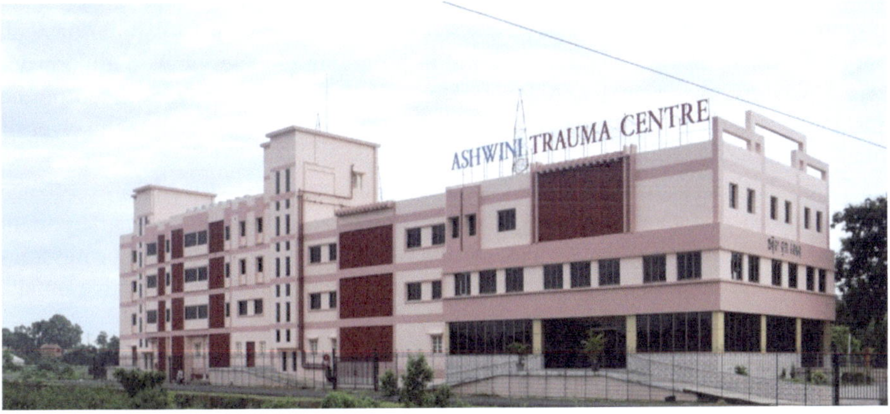

13.1 History of the Center

Ashwini Hospital, located in Cuttack, was established on January 26, 2006, with the vision to provide quality healthcare services to the community. Over the years, the hospital has achieved significant milestones and played a pivotal role in the healthcare sector. In 2007, Ashwini Hospital collaborated with Smile Train, an NGO dedicated to cleft lip and palate treatment, to provide specialized cleft services to patients. This partnership marked a significant step toward enhancing the hospital's services and expanding its reach to a wider population in need. Another important milestone was the establishment of Ashwini Trauma Centre in 2019, which further

D. Sybil (✉)
Department of Oral Surgery, Faculty of Dentistry, Jamia Millia Islamia, New Delhi, India

S. K. Jena · S. Das · S. K. Das · S. Mahakud · S. Shirin
Smile Train Cleft Centre, Ashwini Hospital, Cuttack, India

P. Batra et al. (eds.), *The Cleft Care Framework in India*,
https://doi.org/10.1007/978-981-99-8968-3_13

strengthened the hospital's capabilities to handle emergency cases and provide comprehensive trauma care.

Dr. Subrat Kumar Jena, the Chairman of Ashwini Hospital, and Dr. Maya Gantayet, the Managing Director, have been the driving forces behind the center's success and growth. Their leadership and dedication to improving healthcare services have earned the hospital a strong reputation in the region.

Ashwini Hospital has received support from various funding agencies to sustain and expand its operations. The principal funding agencies include Biju Swasthya Kalyan Yojana (BSKY), the State Health Scheme of Odisha, which aims to provide accessible healthcare to all residents of the state. The hospital also receives support from the Central Government Health Scheme (CGHS) and the Employees' State Insurance Corporation (ESIC), ensuring healthcare coverage for government employees and insured workers, respectively. Furthermore, the collaboration with Smile Train NGO has been instrumental in providing cleft services to underprivileged patients. Additionally, Ashwini Hospital participates in various corporate insurance schemes, which enable a broader range of patients to avail themselves of quality healthcare services.

Throughout its history, Ashwini Hospital has continuously strived for excellence in healthcare delivery, expanding its infrastructure, achieving landmark patient numbers, and enhancing its services. With its dedicated team of medical professionals and commitment to patient care, the center continues to make a positive impact on the health and well-being of the community it serves.

13.2 Present Scenario of the Center

The center is currently headed by Dr. Subrat Kumar Jena. The team at the center consists of several doctors, surgeons, clinicians, and support staff. The doctors include Dr. Ruchi Gupta (Plastic Surgeon), Dr. Shibani Das (Maxillofacial Surgeon), Dr. Rashmi Ranjan Satapathy (Anesthesiologist), Dr. Surya Kanta Das (Orthodontist), Dr. Lara Mishra (General Dentist), and Dr. Niranjan Mohanty (Pediatrician). The center also has Ms. Shubhasmita Mahakud (Speech and Language therapist), Ms. Swaleha Shirin (Nutritionist), Mr. Dipti Ranjan Pradhan (Manager Smile Train), and Mr. Tapas Ranjan Acharya (Deputy Manager Smile Train) as part of the team. The nursing team consists of Ms. Subhashree Sahoo, Ms. Madhusmita Mohanty, Ms. Gayatri Sahoo, Ms. Laxmipriya Kandi, Ms. Kumudini, and Ms. Manasi Gayal. The OT team includes Mr. Asit Kumar Nayak, Ms. Ritarani Nayak, Ms. Sasmita Sahoo, Ms. Smruti Rekha, Mr. Gyana, Mr. Bapuji, and Ms. Santilata Sethy.

To date, the center has successfully operated on 7500 cases. The center offers a range of services including surgical services, rehabilitation services, and diagnostic services. The surgical services provided by the center include lip surgery, palate surgery, alveolar bone grafting, fistula closure, palate lengthening, VPI correction (to be started), orthognathic surgery (cases under preparation), cleft rhinoplasty, and distraction osteogenesis. The rehabilitation services offered include speech therapy, orthodontics, nasoalveolar molding, general dentistry, nutritionist services, and counseling. The center also provides diagnostic services such as dental radiography, computed tomography, 2D echocardiography, nasoendoscopy, and videofluoroscopy (services to be started soon).

13.3 Workflow

The workflow system at the center involves a structured process for patient care. During the first visit to the hospital, the child is seen by the surgeon and thoroughly examined. The child's weight is compared with WHO standards, and if necessary, the child is enrolled in the Nutritional program. Children with a complete cleft lip who report to the center within the first few weeks of life are encouraged for NAM treatment. After completing the NAM treatment or achieving age-appropriate weight, the primary lip surgery is performed, which typically requires a minimum of three months and 5 kg of weight. The primary palate surgery is performed at a minimum of 9 months of age and 9 kg of weight. Speech counseling starts immediately after 1 month of palate surgery and continues as advised by the therapist. If a patient requires primary cleft surgeries but does not have the appropriate weight according to WHO standards, they are sent for nutritional counseling, and the surgery is performed only after the child achieves the appropriate weight.

Pre-SABG orthodontics begins at 6 years of age. SABG surgery is done during the canine eruption phase, followed by post-SABG orthodontics. Lip revision and rhinoplasty surgeries are generally carried out after the age of 16, but in cases of failed primary cleft repairs, they can be considered at an earlier time. The center has also started orthodontically preparing appropriate cases for orthognathic surgery, and these surgeries will be performed soon. Additionally, the center provides treatment to cleft patients who were not primarily treated at their center based on their requirements and complaints.

The center faces several challenges, including inadequate funding for cleft children needing surgeries beyond cleft repair and higher investigations. The instability of doctors, clinicians, and support staff is another challenge. Managing patient flow is also a challenge that the center faces. Despite these challenges, the center strives to provide comprehensive care to cleft patients and improve their quality of life.

13.4 Clinical Protocol

At the center, the preferred surgical techniques for unilateral cleft lip are Millard's Rotation advancement technique or the Modified Millard's technique, while for bilateral cleft lip Millard's Mulliken technique is used. When it comes to primary cleft palate, Von Langenbeck technique and Bardach's two-flap palatoplasty technique along with Intra Velar Veloplasty are preferred. The average duration of hospital stay for primary surgeries is typically around 2–3 days for cleft lip and 3–4 days for cleft palate. Sutures in lip surgeries are generally removed between 10 and 15 days after the procedure. The follow-up system at the center is comprehensive and includes various aspects. Suture removal for lip surgeries takes place within the aforementioned timeframe. Follow-up appointments for palate surgeries are scheduled after 1 month, while SABG is evaluated after 15 days. Additionally, patients are enrolled in a nutritional program on a monthly basis. Speech follow-up sessions are offered as advised by therapists and orthodontic follow-up appointments as recommended by the clinician.

The center provides various support services to the patients. These include accommodation for patients and their attenders, transport allowances and food services to ensure their comfort and convenience throughout their treatment journey.

13.5 Community Outreach

The center primarily serves the regions of western Odisha and Coastal Odisha. To reach needy patients, it employs several methods. They receive referrals from primary healthcare centers, organize cleft camps to identify and treat patients, and rely on the positive word of mouth to spread awareness about the center and its services.

The center actively engages in community-based services through collaborations with government agencies and primary health centers. In particular, it works closely with the RBSK (Rashtriya Bal Swasthya Karyakram) teams in various districts and has also partnered with the Chirantan NGO, which assists in identifying cleft patients in rural areas, enabling the center to extend support and services to those in need.

13.6 Academic and Research Activities

The center has been actively engaged in various academic and research activities focused on cleft care. In terms of funded research projects, the center is currently conducting several ongoing studies. These projects include a prospective study on the dental and skeletal development of children with and without complete unilateral cleft lip and palate, a split-mouth three-dimensional study comparing the stage of canine root formation and eruption path in unilateral cleft lip and palate children, and an investigation into the analgesic efficacy at the donor site after bone harvest from the iliac crest in patients undergoing alveolar bone grafting surgery.

In addition to these research projects, the center has made significant contributions through scientific papers. Some notable publications include papers on subjective assessment of nasolabial appearance in patients treated with or without primary rhinoplasty, orthodontic preparation in cleft patients, orthodontic cleft work in the mixed dentition period, and the burden of orofacial clefts based on the center's experience in a low-income state in India. Furthermore, the center has presented research findings on feeding challenges in newborn babies with cleft palate deformity and innovative approaches to enhance nutritional delivery as well as studies on lip taping efficacy, subjective evaluation of nasolabial esthetics in operated cases of complete cleft lip and palate, and the fabrication of an anatomical nipple for cleft palate babies.

One of the important contributions of the center to cleft care is a patent granted by the Government of India for the development of an anatomical nipple designed specifically for cleft palate babies. This patent, pioneered by Dr. Surya Kanta Das, signifies the center's commitment to addressing the unique challenges faced by infants with cleft palate deformities and their nutritional needs. Overall, the center's extensive research activities and innovative solutions demonstrate its dedication to advancing cleft care and improving the quality of life for affected individuals.

13.7 Future Direction

Ashwini Hospital strives to establish a world-class institute in healthcare and stay at the forefront of medical technology and best practices. The hospital aims to fulfill the long-felt need for true super-speciality healthcare in the region. By focusing on continuous improvement and innovation, the hospital aims to set new standards in patient care, medical education, and research.

To the next generation of cleft care personnel, the message from Ashwini Hospital is to holistically treat the cleft child. This entails not only addressing the physical aspect of the cleft condition through surgical interventions but also considering the psychological, social, and emotional well-being of the child.

For future cleft centers, Ashwini Hospital recommends incorporating various specialties to provide holistic and comprehensive cleft care. Cleft conditions often require multidisciplinary approaches, involving experts from fields such as plastic surgery, orthodontics, speech therapy, audiology, psychology, and social work. By establishing collaborative teams of specialists, cleft centers can ensure that patients receive comprehensive care that addresses all aspects of their condition, leading to better outcomes and improved patient satisfaction.

In India, cleft care currently lacks awareness, comprehensive care, and adequate funds. Many people in the country are still unaware of cleft conditions, their causes, and the available treatment options. This leads to delays in seeking medical help, which can negatively impact the outcomes for cleft patients. Furthermore, comprehensive cleft care involves numerous interventions including surgery, speech therapy, dental care, and psychosocial support, which is not widely accessible or affordable for all individuals in India. Finally, there is a need for increased funding to support research, training programs, and infrastructure development in the field of cleft care. Addressing these challenges is pivotal to improving the quality of cleft care in India and ensuring that all individuals affected by cleft conditions receive the support and treatment they need.

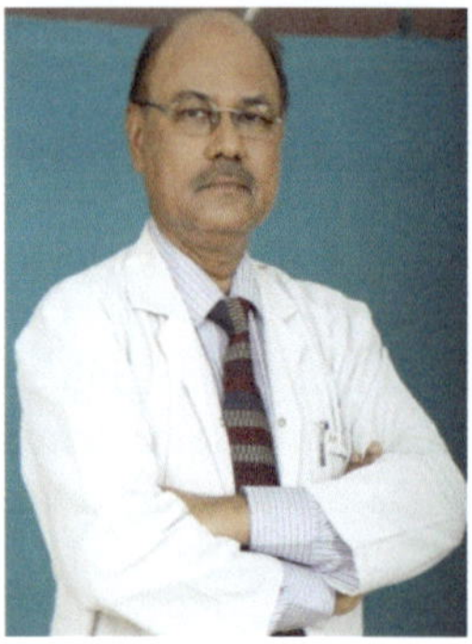

Dr. Subrat Kumar Jena (Plastic surgeon)

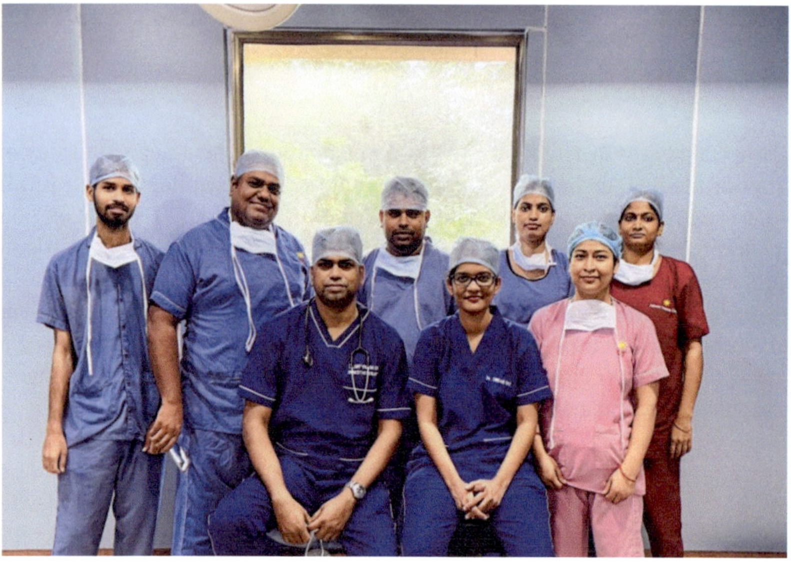

Cleft Care team at Ashwini Hospital

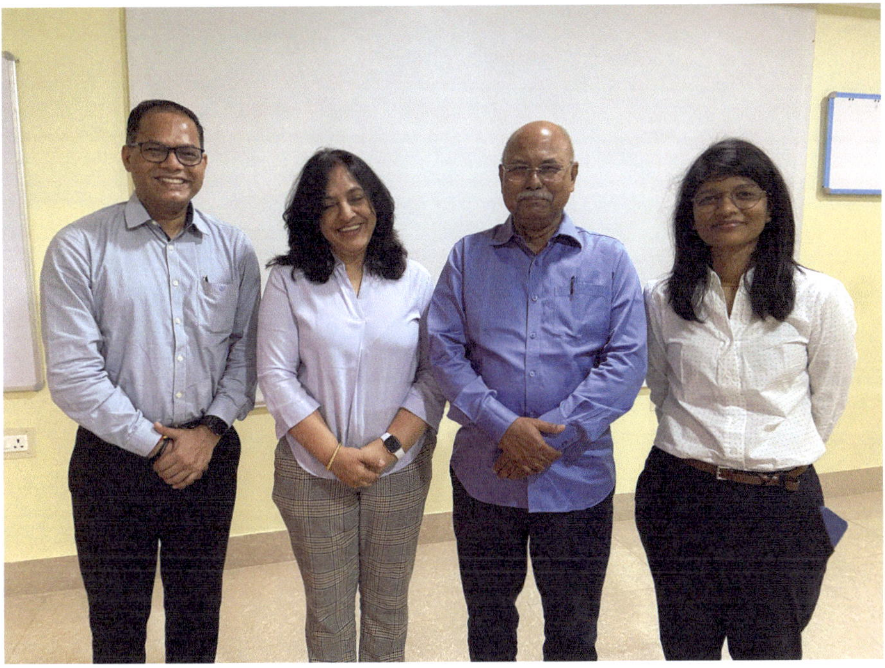

From right to left - Prof. Surya Kanta Das (Orthodontist) Ms. Leela Imam (Senior Director-Education & Training and Comprehensive Cleft Care Programs; Smile train) Dr. Subrat Jena (Plasic Surgeon and Director) Dr. Shibani Das (Oral Surgeon)

Part V
The West India Experience

Chapter 14
Global Hospital and Research Center, Mt. Abu, Rajasthan

Puneet Batra and Sharad Mehta

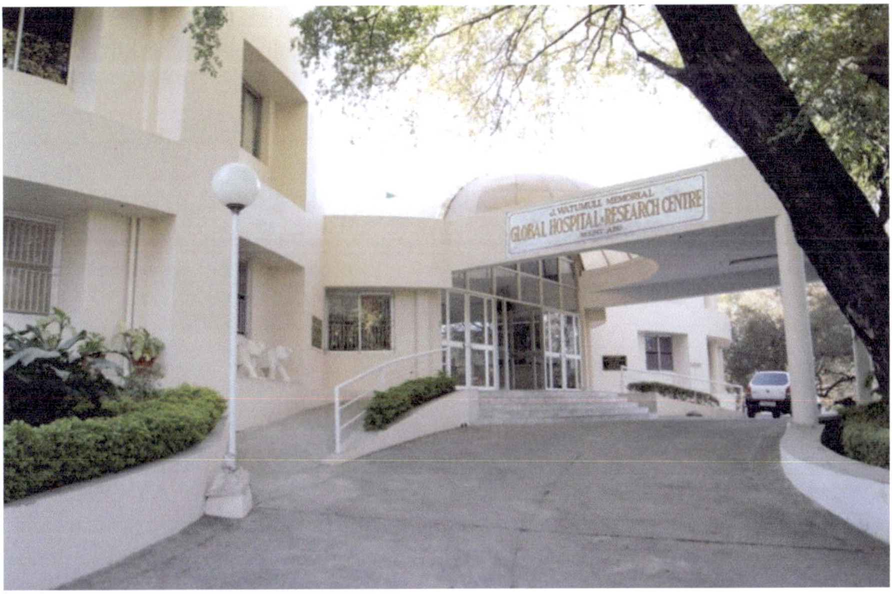

14.1 History of the Center

Cleft and Craniofacial Center Unit in Global Hospital and Research Center, established in 2001, has made significant strides since its inception. Under the guidance of its pioneer, Dr. Jan Lilja and Dr. Shailesh Vadodaria, the hospital has become one of the world class healthcare facilities in Mt Abu, Rajasthan.

In the past, the center has achieved various important milestones in cleft care. In 2001, Great Ormond Street Hospital (GOSH) with Dr. Michael Mars, Dr. Sujata

P. Batra (✉) · S. Mehta
Global Hospital, Mount Abu, Rajasthan, India

P. Batra et al. (eds.), *The Cleft Care Framework in India*,
https://doi.org/10.1007/978-981-99-8968-3_14

Kelkar, Dr. Brian Sommarlad, and Dr. Puneet Batra conducted a cleft camp. In 2004, Dr. Sharad Mehta (ENT surgeon) started doing regular cleft surgeries. In 2008, Dr. Partha Sadhu joined as plastic surgeon in Smile train program alongside speech therapist and orthodontist. In 2016, Dr. Gopal Krishna joined the center as Director of Smile Train Program. Then, after 2 years, Dr. Ayyappan Thangavel from Ahemdabad joined as Director of Smile train program. In 2018, Dr. Keyur Mevada, Oral surgeon also joined the program, enhancing the center's capabilities to address a wider range of surgical treatment procedures in cleft patients. The center's commitment to the excellence is further highlighted by its affiliation with Smile Train, one of the principal funding agencies. This center has almost all the necessary resources, enabling it to provide high-quality care to the patients in need. Over the years, the hospital has also received support from other secondary funding agencies which helped in reinforcing its ability to deliver the comprehensive dental and medical services.

Since its establishment, Cleft and Craniofacial center has continually evolved, both in terms of its infrastructure and the availability of care. It owes its success not only to its founder but also to CMO Dr. Pratap Midha along with the succeeding doctors and personnel who have played key roles in shaping the center's development and improvement. With a rich history and a commitment to compassionate care it is serving in Southwest Rajasthan.

14.2 Present Scenario of the Center

Currently, Dr. Sharad Mehta is the lead ENT Surgeon. Alongside him, the center has a dedicated team of doctors, surgeons, clinicians, and support staff who contribute to the successful operation of the center. The doctors in the team include Dr. Puneet Batra as Orthodontist and Dr. Akash Jain as Orthodontist and visiting Speech Therapist.

The center has performed a substantial number of surgeries over the years, with a total of around 2500 cases operated till now. To provide proper care to the patients, the center has a wide range of services. The surgical procedures available for patients are innumerable such as primary lip repair surgery, palatal repair surgery, primary and secondary alveolar bone grafting, all types of fistula closure, palate lengthening, velopharyngeal incompetence correction, orthognathic surgery, cleft rhinoplasty, and distraction osteogenesis. The center provides services along with surgical procedures such as naso-alveolar molding, speech therapy, audiometry, orthodontics, general dentistry, nutritional services, psychiatric counseling, and ENT services. The center has availability to the diagnostic aids such as dental radiography (OPG and lateral cephalograms), cone beam computed tomography, 2D echocardiography, nasoendoscopy, and videofluoroscopy.

Workflow The workflow system at the center follows a comprehensive approach. Upon referral, newborns are initially examined by the Orthodontist for PSIO if required. After this, the case is reviewed in the joint clinic and then planned for lip repair in consultation with nutritionist, pediatrician, and anesthetists. Lip surgery is usually done at the age of 4–5 months and palatal repair is done at 9–12 months. The speech therapy provided in the age group of 2–5 years when it is crucially required. In the mixed dentition period, the cleft patients needing orthodontic treatment to prepare for primary alveolar bone graft and maxillary protraction is provided. Corrective orthodontic treatment is done after permanent dentition has erupted. Some of the patients are operated for orthognathic surgery after cessation of growth with the help of orthodontics.

Despite its success, the center faces several challenges. Inadequate funding poses a significant obstacle, making it difficult to meet the growing demands and maintain high-quality services. The center also experiences challenges related to the stability of doctors, clinicians, and support staff, which may affect the continuity of patient care. Managing patient flow efficiently is another concern for the center. Additionally, patient follow-up presents a challenge, requiring dedicated efforts to ensure comprehensive care and monitoring beyond the initial treatment. Overcoming these challenges will enable the center to continue providing excellent care to their patients.

14.3 Clinical Protocol

The preferred surgical techniques for at the center are Modified Millards repair for lip correction and Furlows repair with primary buccal flaps for palate repair.

For the primary surgeries, the average duration of admission for a patient at our center is typically 2–3 days. This duration may vary depending on the specific requirements and the progress of the patient's recovery. In the case of lip repair surgery, suture removal is typically scheduled after 7–10 days. This allows the wound to heal in sufficient time and ensures its proper closure. For cleft palate patients, the center has a follow-up period of every 4 weeks, during which their recovery is closely monitored. On the other hand, cleft lip patients are typically followed up for 10 days to ensure proper healing and address any concerns. Additionally, patients who are nutritionally deficient or anemic are scheduled for monthly follow-ups to assess their nutritional status and provide necessary interventions. Apart from these specific cases, regular appointments are scheduled based on the individual treatment protocol devised for each patient.

Patient and attender accommodation, transport allowance, food services, rehabilitation services are all offered by the center.

14.4 Community Outreach

This center focuses on serving the Southwest Rajasthan and reaches out to needy patients through various means. Referrals from primary healthcare centers enable this center to identify patients who require specialized services. Cleft camps are also conducted by the center in nearby suburban and rural areas. Also, the center actively engage in door-to-door campaigns in slums and rural areas, where their team visits the communities to raise awareness about cleft lip and palate procedures and explain treatment information about their services and other facilities. The center's popularity is through word of mouth has also been instrumental in reaching out to those who require their services.

14.5 Academic and Research Activities

One of the notable achievements is the development of yardstick, i.e., "Use of Bauru Yardstick in Patients with Complete Bilateral Cleft Lip and Palate at an Indian Center" at our center.

14.6 Future Direction

The center aims to provide the team support for the interdisciplinary approach with the help of comprehensive care specialists and providing the best of technological and research innovation support with a human touch at affordable prices. The next generation of cleft care personnel, the center emphasizes the importance of hard work and patience in achieving success in this specialized field.

In the context of cleft care in India, the lack of comprehensive cleft care teams has always been a significant challenge. However, the landscape is evolving, and we are witnessing a positive change with the increasing number of dedicated specialists committed to providing comprehensive cleft care. By fostering the collaboration among various specialists, including surgeons, orthodontists, speech therapists, psychologists, and social workers, holistic care for every patient can be ensured. Through continued efforts, there is a hope to bridge this gap and ensure that every individual with a cleft condition receives the best possible care and support.

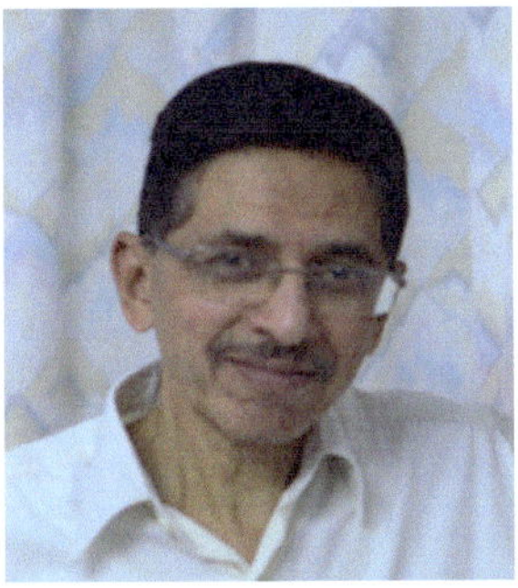

Dr. Sharad Mehta (Plastic Surgeon)

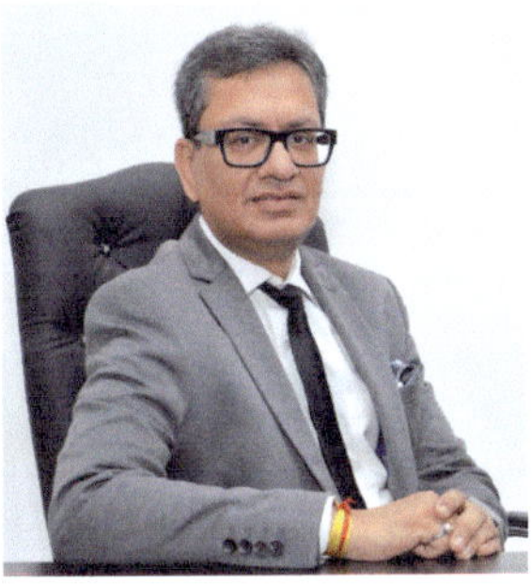

Dr. Puneet Batra (Orthodontist)

Part VI
The South India Experience

Chapter 15
GSR Institute of Craniomaxillofacial and Facial Plastic Surgery, Hyderabad, Telangana

Badri Thiruvenkatachari, Srinivas Gosla Reddy, Rajgopal R. Reddy, and Avni Pande

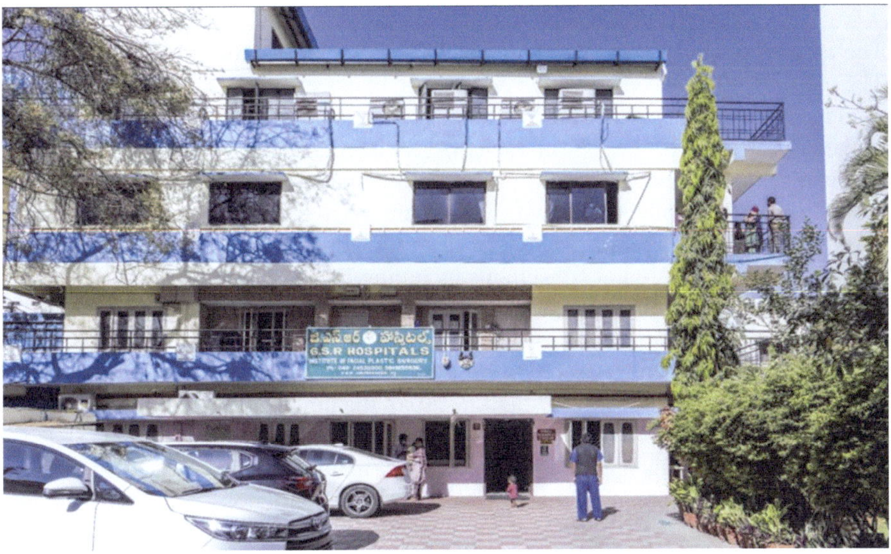

B. Thiruvenkatachari (✉)
Dental Research, Sree Balaji Medical College and Hospital, The Cleft and Craniofacial Centre, Chennai, India

S. G. Reddy · R. R. Reddy · A. Pande
GSR Institute of Craniomaxillofacial and Facial Plastic Surgery, Hyderabad, Telangana, India

P. Batra et al. (eds.), *The Cleft Care Framework in India*,
https://doi.org/10.1007/978-981-99-8968-3_15

15.1 History

GSR Institute of Craniofacial and Facial Plastic Surgery (GSRICFS), a state of art hospital situated in Hyderabad came into being in October 1996 as a specialized centre dedicated to providing comprehensive care for individuals with craniofacial and facial plastic surgery needs. Founded by Dr. Srinivas Gosla Reddy (also the centre head), the centre has since become a renowned institution in the field, serving the needs for all congenital facial surgeries primarily in the south and central parts of India. While, Dr. Srinivas Gosla Reddy, Dr. Rajgopal Reddy, and Dr. Avni Pandey are the pioneers of the centre, these along with Dr. Ashish Fanan, Dr. Madhav Thumati, and Dr. Heena Syed have played a pivotal role in the centre.

15.2 Present Scenario

The centre operates under the Hyderabad Cleft Society, a non-profit organization. The medical advisory board which consists of 13 esteemed doctors from around the world speaks volumes about the institute's dedication to maintaining high standards of patient care. With experts from the USA, Switzerland, Italy, France, Netherlands, Germany, and Europe, the board brings diverse perspectives and expertise to the table. Institute has collaborated with 16 institutions in India and Europe for research and training. GSRICFS is a 50 bedded hospital with two state-of-the-art operation theatres. There are six chief consultants including Dr. Gosla Reddy and four fellows working along with other 50 ground staff. GSRICFS has reached key milestones and experienced extraordinary growth, both in terms of infrastructure development and the number of patients served, throughout its journey. The centre has worked constantly to improve its services and maintain the highest levels of patient care.

Infrastructure Development: In its attempt to improve patient care, GSRICFS installed advanced medical equipment in 2005, including Boyle's Machine (Datex Ohmeda), defibrillators, monitors, and an Engstrom ventilator.

In the consequent years, the centre expanded its facilities with cutting-edge technology such as O T Lights (Steris IDS), O T Tables (Healthcare IDS), microscopes (Zeiss), endoscopes (Storz, Pentax), cautery (L & T, SKANRAY, BIONIX), ventilator (GE RE 860), oscillating saw (Stryker), generator (Kirloskar), and a horizontal autoclave (CISCO).

Number of patients operated: 5000 patients were successfully operated upon in the years from 1996 to 2000. Another 5000 patients were surgically treated from 2001 to 2004, 25000 patients from 2005 to 2022, and a whopping 35000 patients have been operated upon till date thereby displaying the centre's devotion and dedication in serving the population.

Services offered: GSRICFS provides a broad range of services to meet the patients' diverse needs. Lip, palate, and fistula closure surgeries have been available since 1996 and alveolar bone grafting started at the centre in 1997. While VPI correction, orthognathic surgery and distraction osteogenesis have been available since 2005, palate lengthening surgery and cleft rhinoplasty have been accessible since 2006 which allowed the centre to achieve phenomenal outcomes in addition to fine-tuning the approaches.

Apart from the surgical services, the centre provides rehabilitation services too. General dentistry, counselling and ENT (Grommet) services are into place since 1996. It also been providing orthodontics, audiometry, and speech therapy since 2001, psychologist since 2005, nutritionist since 2021, and nasoalveolar moulding since 2022.

The services are not just limited to surgical and rehabilitation, advanced diagnostic services are also available since 1996 which include dental radiography, computed tomography, 2D echocardiography. Nasoendoscopy and videfluroscopy have also been made available since 2006.

15.3 Workflow

Global Surgery and Research Institute for Cleft Surgeries has a distinctive workflow system that operates on a hybrid model of blended finance convergence. It generates revenues through collaborations with NGOs and offers free or low-cost surgeries to patients from low socioeconomic backgrounds. The philosophy is to create, collaborate, and cooperate in order to deliver healthcare services to those in need. GSRICFS believes that charity is not for pity but for the corporatization of health care delivery for needy patients. Through standardization, and engineering surgeries for high volume production, the centre strives to achieve cost-effectiveness and efficiency. GSRICFS is therefore a paradigm of economically healthy entrepreneurship and healthcare innovation. The sliding-scale fee payment system and funding by NGOs are the two main sources of revenue. Collaborations with NGOs involved in clefts provide for about 65% of the centre's revenue, while the other 45% comes from affluent patients who pay for the surgeries though the high surgical standards remain the same for all patients. These streams allow the centre to continue its practice of providing free or low-cost surgeries to the impoverished populations. GSRICFS has been instrumental in affecting cultural behavioural patterns and social structures in India. While the patients are encouraged to actively interact and participate in the healthcare delivery process, thereby fostering a sense of ownership and empowerment, the doctors at the same time are encouraged to take on more responsibility and dedication while motivating patients to become active participants in their treatments. The centre relies on funding from organizations such as Smile Train, CCI, Future Faces, Enable, Ravi Foundation, Raj Choudhary Foundation, Sterling Trust, and others.

The centre does face challenges related to unstable human resources, which can impact the continuity of services.

15.4 Clinical Protocol

The centre prefers to use morphofunctional approach for primary cheiloplasty and primary palatoplasty which takes care of the anatomical as well as the functional aspects of lip and palate. On an average, patients undergoing primary surgeries typically require a short hospital stay of 1–2 days. Sutures are removed 15 days post lip surgeries which enables adequate healing, lowers the risk of complications and ensures that the patient's recovery progresses smoothly and uneventfully. The centre follows an organized follow-up system to monitor patients' progress. The follow-up visits are scheduled at specific intervals, including 15 days, 1 month, 6 months, and yearly. However, the exact duration between follow-up visits may vary depending on individual patient needs and the specific procedure performed. Patient and attender accommodation, food services, rehabilitation services, transport services are also provided by the centre.

15.5 Community Outreach

GSRICFS has a wide area of reach in providing free treatment for cleft and craniofacial deformities. Besides the core services, the centre has implemented REACH (Rural Effective, Affordable Comprehensive Healthcare) programme formulated by Dr. Gosla Reddy, that works in slums, schools and communities, and caters to patients from the lower socioeconomic strata by supporting them through treatment, counselling, removing stigma, and fulfilling patient care needs. Nearly 35000 free surgeries and support is provided to more than 100 cleft and congenital orphan kids. The centre reaches patients through various channels such as door-to-door awareness campaigns, referrals from primary health care centres, cleft camps, the centre's popularity, NGOs, and social media. Collaborations with government agencies, primary health centres, and organizations such as FCN (Foundation for Children in Need), RBSK (Rashtriya Bal Swasthya Karyakram), and SACRED camp help GSRICFS to offer free treatment to patients with cleft deformities.

15.6 Academic and Research Activities

GSRICFS is well-known for its outstanding research initiatives in a variety of fields related to cleft and craniofacial conditions. It offers Ph.D. and fellowship programmes through its collaborative research programme with six national and international universities, attracting scholars and researchers from all over the world. Because of its cutting-edge curriculum and advanced infrastructure, the programme has been recognized as a training institute for postgraduate students by 16 universities in India. Dr. GSR, a renowned maxillofacial surgeon, was among the first to be invited to Radboud University in Europe for Ph.D. research. He has made noteworthy contributions to the field and designed his own surgical technique for the treatment of cleft lip and palate, known as the morphofunctional technique, which has received international acclaim. Dr. GSR is an enthusiastic teacher who has trained more than 300 fellows from all over the world. He serves as the chief mentor of the International Association of Oral and Maxillofacial Surgeons and the AO in India in GSRICFS. GSR Hospital is one of the only two institutes recognized by both IAOMFS and AO. Each year, the fellowship programme at GSRICFS trains six promising surgeons, providing them with invaluable skills and knowledge. He is also visiting faculty in more than 10 institutes of India and Europe. Every year nearly 100 post graduate residents visit GSR hospital to learn cleft as a part of their residency programme. Dr. GSR's students revere him and enthusiastically spread his surgical philosophy throughout the world. As a result, his fellows and residents can be found working in almost every state in India and Europe, making a significant contribution to the field of cleft and craniofacial surgery. Dr. GSR has 70 articles to his name and has received various research grants from prestigious organizations such as the Indian Council of Medical Research (ICMR) among others. Through its PhD programmes, the centre has actively contributed to research and education. Several researchers are pursuing PhDs under the supervision of Dr. GSR and other distinguished professionals. These programmes cover a variety of cleft care and related topics, such as surgical techniques, genetic and epigenetic factors, risk factors, health-seeking behaviour, and implant evaluation. These initiatives ensure a steady flow of new information and advances in the field.

Dr. GSR's Cleft School Project exemplifies his charitable spirit and dedication to improving the lives of cleft-affected children. Nearly 100 orphaned or semi-orphaned cleft children from low socioeconomic backgrounds benefit from free housing, education, and support through the project. These children receive a high-quality education in reputed English-medium schools, with all expenses covered by Dr. GSR's trust. The project has been running for 15 years, and some of the children have gone on to pursue PhDs and successful careers. He provides decent living to all his cleft school project students and gives them a safe atmosphere. Not only that, his 60% staff are all cleft and congenital deformities patients.

GSRICFS has actively engaged in fruitful partnerships and research endeavours with numerous medical establishments, at domestic as well as international levels, with the aim of advancing craniofacial and facial plastic surgery. These collaborative efforts have tremendously facilitated the exchange of ideas and expertise, sharing of best approaches and practices, and conducting groundbreaking research in the field of cleft care.

15.7 Future Direction

Dr. GSR's future vision is rooted in the belief that finances should never hinder access to optimal and quality healthcare and he has taken proactive steps to realize this vision by collaborating with different organizations from the USA, Europe, and

India. The centre's motto is that no patient should ever be denied treatment due to financial constraints. Future generations should be well trained in Cleft care through clinical programmes that emphasize collaboration, sustainability, meeting local needs, and appropriate process considerations. The future looks bright for GSRICFS, and the centre is looking to train more and more young surgeons, particularly from northern and eastern India, where comprehensive cleft centres are scarce. This vision must lay emphasis on knowledge application and allow for the evaluation of intended outcomes. The importance of a clear vision in achieving this cannot be overlooked. Core values and principles can also serve as a backdrop for competencies and if the Institute's concepts are adopted by its trainees, a fairer society will definitely emerge.

Cleft surgery involves sophisticated infrastructure, instrumentation, specialized anaesthetists, and high ended post-operative care, as well as collaboration among surgeons, anaesthetists, paediatricians, psychologists, orthodontists, and specialist nurses. In a developing nation like India, acquiring all of these facilities and performing cleft surgeries requires a significant amount of effort to establish and develop. If the Institute's concepts are adopted by its trainees a better future is a certainty. Until then, let us create, collaborate, and collaborate in the fight against these dreadful deformities that not only cause functional problems but also psychologically cripple patients.

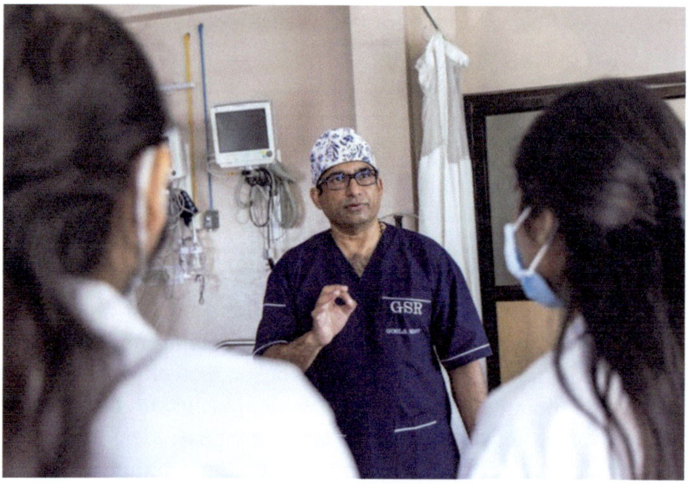

Dr.Srinivas Gosla Reddy – Director of GSR Hospital and Surgeon (Case Discussion)

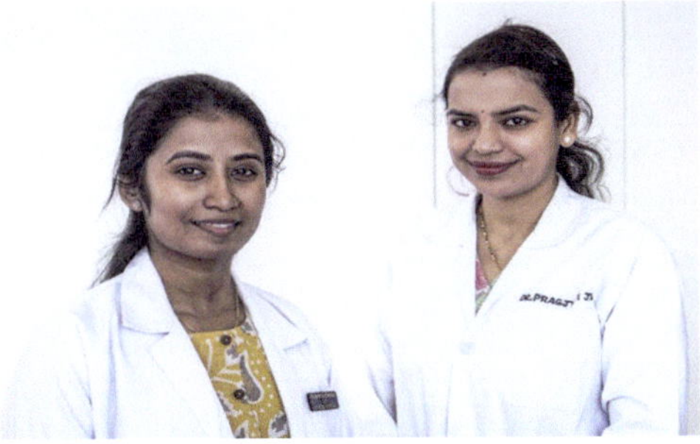

Dr. Myrtle Ciphora (Speech Therapist) and Dr Pragjyoti Jha (Dental surgeon)

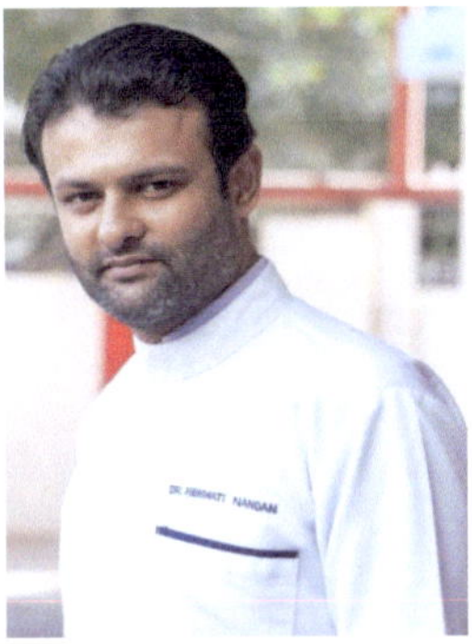

Dr. Hemwati Nandan (Orthodontist)

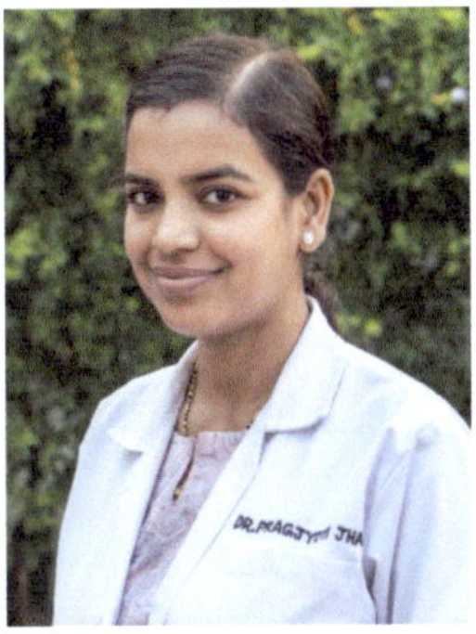

Dr. Pragjyoti Jha (Dental Surgeon)

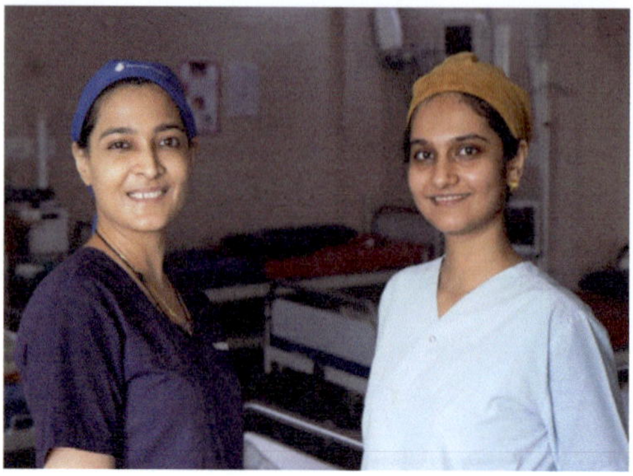

Dr. Avni Pandey and Dr. Heena Sayed (Consultants – Surgeons)

Chapter 16
Cleft Leadership Centre, Bhagwan Mahaveer Jain Hospital, Bengaluru, Karnataka

Panchali Batra, Pritham Shetty, Krishnamurthy Bonanthaya, Dipesh Rao, V. S. Aparna, Namrata, Arvind Sivakumar, Shruti Bijapur, Mansi Puranik, and Priyal Sheth Mehta

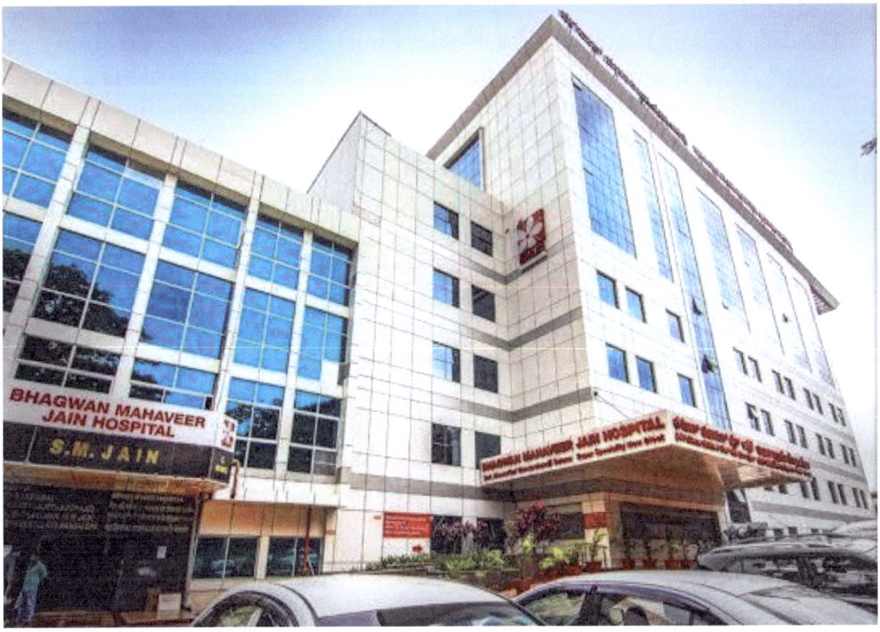

P. Batra (✉)
Department of Orthodontics, Faculty of Dentistry, Jamia Millia Islamia, New Delhi, India
e-mail: p.batra@jmi.ac.in

P. Shetty · K. Bonanthaya · D. Rao · V. S. Aparna · Namrata · A. Sivakumar · S. Bijapur · M. Puranik · P. S. Mehta
CLC, Smile Train at Bhagwan Mahaveer Jain Hospital, Bangalore, India

P. Batra et al. (eds.), *The Cleft Care Framework in India*,
https://doi.org/10.1007/978-981-99-8968-3_16

16.1 History of the Center

The Smile Train Cleft Leadership Centre, located in Bangalore, India, has a rich history marked by significant milestones and the dedication of exceptional individuals. Established in May 2005, the center has become a pioneering institution in the field of cleft lip and palate surgeries. Dr. Krishnamurthy Bonanthaya, a visionary surgeon, played a crucial role as the founder and pioneer of the center. His unwavering commitment and expertise laid the foundation for the center's success. In 2013, Dr. Pritham Shetty joined Dr. Bonanthaya. Pritham Shetty was with the centre from day 1 in may 2005 as the second surgeon and has since played an instrumental role in performing cleft surgeries. Additionally, Dr. Aparna, a speech and language pathologist, joined the unit full-time in 2013, and Dr. Renu Parmar, an orthodontist, joined in 2012, both contributing significantly to the center's comprehensive care approach.

The center has undergone remarkable infrastructural development over the years. In August 2020, it moved from a modest ground-floor facility consisting of two rooms to a spacious sixth-floor facility with six dedicated rooms. This expansion provided an improved environment for patient care and enhanced the center's capacity to treat more individuals with cleft conditions.

Throughout its history, the Smile Train Cleft Leadership Centre has achieved several notable milestones. From its inception, the center has been dedicated to providing high-quality cleft surgeries and comprehensive care to patients. With the support of Smile Train, a prominent funding agency, and additional financial assistance from the Hospital, the center has been able to offer its services to a significant number of patients, improving their quality of life and restoring their smiles.

The Smile Train Cleft Leadership Centre in Bangalore continues to be a beacon of hope for individuals with cleft conditions. With a strong foundation built by Dr. Bonanthaya and the ongoing dedication of Dr. Shetty, Dr. Aparna, Dr. Parmar, and the rest of the team, the center remains at the forefront of cleft care, providing transformative surgeries and comprehensive support to countless individuals and their families.

16.2 Present Scenario of the Center

The center is currently headed by Dr. Pritham Shetty, who also serves as the Project Director. The team consists of various doctors, surgeons, clinicians, and support staff. The surgeons include Dr. Pritham Shetty, Dr. Dipesh Rao, and Dr. Krishnamurthy Bonanthaya himself. Dr. Aparna VS and Ms. Namrtha are the Speech and Language Pathologists, while Dr. Arvind Sivakumar and Dr. Shruti Bijapur are the Orthodontists. Ms. Mansi Puranik is the Nutritionist, Dr. Priyal Sheth Mehta is the Pedodontist, and Ms. Latha is the Psychologist. Miss Madhuri S serves as the Secretary, and the nursing staff includes Sanjana, Jhansi, and Naseema.

Miss Khatija handles the reception duties, and there are also surgical fellows, Dr. Sanjana Kapoor and Dr. Srishti Ghorpade.

Since its establishment, the center has operated on approximately 10,202 cases. The center offers a wide range of services to its patients. In terms of surgical services, they specialize in lip surgery, palate surgery, alveolar bone grafting, fistula closure, palate lengthening, VPI correction, orthognathic surgery, cleft rhinoplasty, and distraction osteogenesis. Rehabilitation services provided by the center include speech therapy, audiometry, orthodontics, nasoalveolar molding, general dentistry, nutritionist consultations, psychological support, counseling, and ENT services such as grommet insertion. Diagnostic services offered include dental radiography, computed tomography, 2D echocardiography, nasoendoscopy, and videofluoroscopy.

16.3 Workflow System

The workflow system at the center begins with the registration and entry of the patient's file into the electronic data system upon arrival. The patients are then initially seen by the surgeons. Based on the specific treatment requirements, the patients are referred to the respective clinicians for further treatment.

One of the main challenges faced by the center is inadequate funding. This poses difficulties in providing comprehensive care, especially for babies requiring additional hospital admissions due to nutritional deficiencies or other reasons. Additional funding would greatly benefit the center by ensuring timely bill payments during such occasions.

16.4 Clinical Protocol

At the center, the average duration of admission for primary surgeries is typically around 2 days. Following the surgery, a well-structured follow-up system is in place to ensure the patient's postoperative care is properly monitored. The patient is scheduled for follow-up appointments at specific intervals, including 7 days, 1 month, and 6 months after the surgery and if there are any specific concerns or requirements, the patient can avail themselves of regular appointments with other specialized care services as needed.

The center also provides various support services to enhance the overall experience and convenience for the patients. The patient and the attender can stay in the ward when admitted for the surgery and during the post op care. Transport allowance is given to patients who cannot afford the charges and need reimbursement. During COVID-19 times all the RT PCRS were also taken care of by Smile train.

16.5 Community Outreach

The center has a wide area of reach, treating patients within a 400-km radius. On few occasions, patients do come from far beyond this radius too.

To reach out to needy patients, various strategies have been employed. Firstly, the center receives referrals from primary healthcare centers, which occasionally involve recommendations from doctors in the neighborhood and surrounding areas. Cleft camps are also conducted in partnership with a group of dedicated social workers. These camps are organized in peri-urban and rural areas, resulting in an average influx of 5–10 patients per month. Another significant contributor to the patient base is the popularity of the center through word of mouth. Patients and parents who have been treated at the center serve as powerful advocates, spreading awareness about the center's services to others. This word of mouth has become the most influential medium for generating patient referrals. Moreover, the center plans to expand its reach further by commissioning a van. This van will cover a 300-km radius, allowing the center to provide teletherapy for speech services and conduct patient screenings. The center is actively seeking collaborations with government agencies and private sector organizations. Currently, one government agency is already in the pipeline for partnership. Although there are no challenges regarding patient flow at present, the center is committed to exploring opportunities to enhance the outreach efforts and support the community.

16.6 Academic and Research Activities

Over the past 10 years, the center has been actively involved in cleft fellowships, training a number of fellows and witnessing their remarkable achievements. The list of Indian fellows includes Kirana Bhat and Dipesh Rao (2010–2011), Mandeep Khokar (2011–2012), Anjani Jha (2012–2013), Vivek Gupta (2013–2014), Sankarshan Chowdari and Saumya Tripathi (2014–2015), Samarat Tawde, Sony Pullan, and Neeti Rajgopalan (2015–2016), Kalhan Ambardar and Neha Abhichandani (2016–2017), Divya Khaunte and Tulasi Nayak (2017–2018), Jazna Jalil and Srinisha Murali (2018–2019), Som Ranjan Pathak and Nikhil Govindan (2019–2020), and Itrat Hussain and Shibasis Biswas (2020–2021). Additionally, the center has also welcomed international fellows such as Mohammed Al-Harthy (2014), Ahmed Maki Merza (2016), Amel (2018), Sahar Nadel and Ashok Dongol (2019). These fellows have made significant contributions to the field of cleft care, enhancing their knowledge and skills to provide better treatment outcomes.

The center's notable contributions in cleft care lie in the comprehensive and holistic approach offered to patients. It ensures that patients receive care across various aspects of their treatment journey, including nutrition, psychology, orthodontics, speech therapy, dentistry, and surgery. By providing all these services under one roof, this center not only offers convenience to patients but also gathers valuable data over the years, enabling the conduction of extensive research and refine best practices in cleft care. The center has also incorporated advanced technologies like CBCT, surgical planning software, intra-oral scanning, and 3D printing into the diagnosis and treatment planning processes, further improving the quality of being delivered.

Cleft, as a difference, is punctuated with socio-economic challenges in India. At the heart of these challenges is the cultural taboo. From a patient's point of view, cleft care in India lacks patients' awareness on whether the difference is treatable, accessibility to the right centers, specialized and dedicated healthcare professionals, hospital infrastructure, and other support mechanisms for supporting cleft patients besides the lack of adequate funding, given that cleft tends to affect patients that are economically disadvantaged more than their wealthier counterparts.

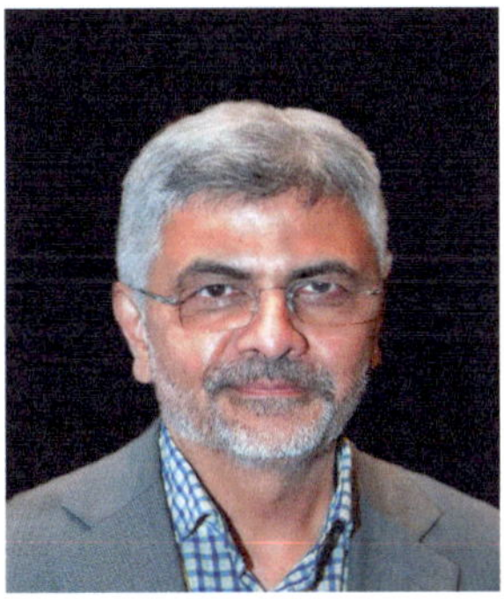

Dr. Krishnamurthy Bonanthaya (Oral and Maxillofacial Surgeon)

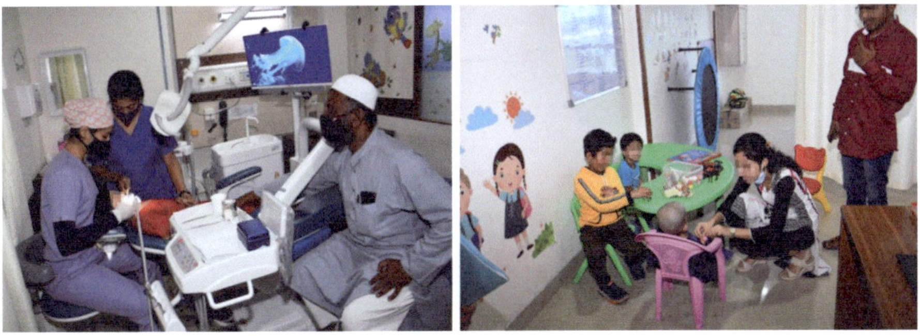

Pediatric care and counseling

Chapter 17
INGA Health Foundation, Bengaluru, Karnataka

Panchali Batra, Krishna Shama Rao, K. Chethana, and Aparajita Shankar

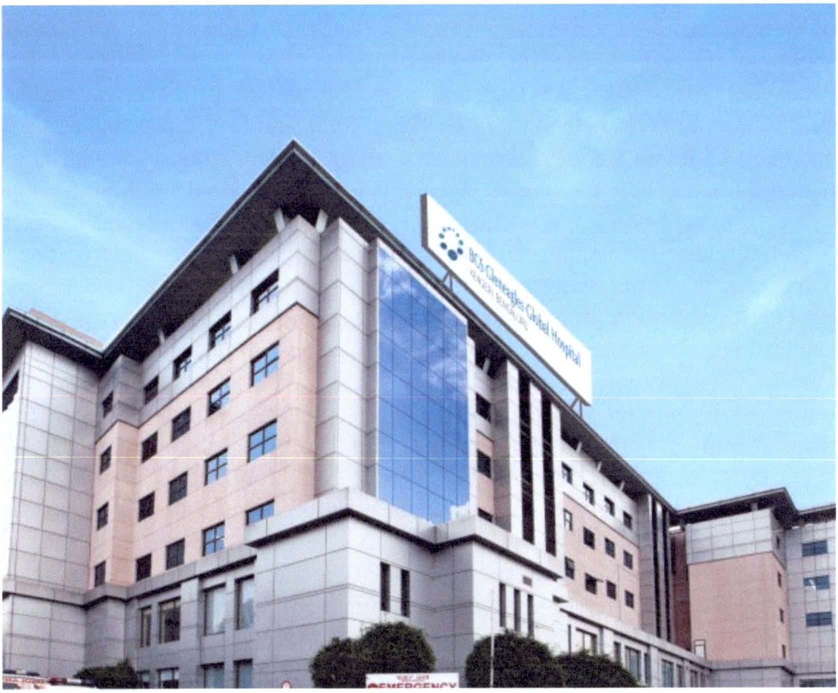

History of the Centre The INGA Health foundation started in the year 2006 by Dr. Krishna Shama Rao (MBBS, FRCS(Ed), BDS, MDS, FDSRCS (Eng)) who is also the Chief Trustee, with the vision of commissioning a comprehensive surgical

P. Batra (✉)
Department of Orthodontics, Faculty of Dentistry, Jamia Millia Islamia, New Delhi, India
e-mail: p.batra@jmi.ac.in

K. S. Rao · K. Chethana · A. Shankar
Craniofacial Centre Inga Health Foundation, Bangalore, India

P. Batra et al. (eds.), *The Cleft Care Framework in India*,
https://doi.org/10.1007/978-981-99-8968-3_17

centre in each Indian state to treat deserving children free, and thereby emerging as a centre of first recall. INGA Health Foundation forged longstanding arrangements with seven hospitals across three states and one union territory (Karnataka, West Bengal, Jharkhand, and J&K).

The foundation has achieved some noteworthy milestones, over the years. After being registered as a trust in 2006–2007, it started centres in Mangalore, Srinagar, and Surat in 2007–2008. The following year saw starting of centres in Bhubaneswar, Mumbai, Vizag, Patna, and Agra and a workshop in Bhubaneswar. In 2009–2010, workshops were conducted in Srinagar, Vizag, and Ahmedabad. The year 2010–2011 witnessed hosting of a conference on craniofacial anomalies in Mangalore, conduction of the first meeting of the newly formed Medical Advisory Board in Chennai, and holding of the annual board meeting in Bangalore.

In the year 2011–2012, the foundation opened second office in Bangalore, launched Project First Smile by the VRT (Vizag Round Table) 77 in Vizag, assisted German Cleft Children's Aid Society with a centre in Bangalore, commenced an international training programme, engaged Ushdev International Limited to adopt Mumbai centre, held first joint meeting with international partner organisations in Hanoi and conducted workshop and annual meet in Patna. It also held biannual board meeting in Patna, sponsored Indocleftcon 2012 event in Bangalore and launched cleft prevention programme in Vizag the same year and was visited by a German business delegation and Dr. Wolfgang Schuster (Lord Mayor, Stuttgart) to mark the 2000th operation in Ahmedabad.

Continuing its progress, in 2012–2013, the foundation launched speech and functional therapy project, got the German Cleft Children's Aid Society to adopt a centre in Coorg, inaugurated a training institute in Bangalore, reopened head office in Bangalore, opened a centre in Noida, completed 7500 surgeries, set up a centre in Bangalore and got separated from German Cleft Children's Aid Society. The first craniofacial surgery funded by Being Human Foundation was completed in 2013–2014. Ushdev International commenced funding of cleft surgeries, 25 craniofacial surgeries were completed and HDFC funded craniofacial operations in the year 2014–2015.

In the subsequent year, the foundation successfully initiated a partnership with Operation Smile USA, one of the largest NGOs in Facial Deformities. Through this partnership, IHF is expected to gain significant insight into large mission programmes. It is an ongoing partnership, with a focus of growing across the nation. Operation Smile, founded in 1982 by Dr. Bill Magee and Kathy Magee with a vision that safe surgery is not a privilege, but a universal human right, focuses on providing safe surgery for those in need. Operation Smile now operates in more than 30 countries and provides world class cleft care by empowering local health professionals through training and education. It also caters the rehabilitation needs of the patients through speech therapy, nutritional support, dentistry, orthodontics, and psychosocial support. Operation Smile supports INGA Health Foundation through Operational Smile India charitable trust and Operational Smile Inc., and also independently operates centres in Durgapur, Siliguri, and Hazirabad.

INGA Health Foundation, in 2016–2017, tied-up with "Department of Health & Family Welfare, Government of Karnataka" formally which led to a MOU between IHF & RBSK hence ensuring that patients from all districts of Karnataka with Craniofacial deformities are identified and referred to the Bangalore centre. In the same year, a medical mission was successfully done in West Bengal in partnership with Operation Smile.

From 2017 to 2018, Oracle commenced funding of cleft, maxillofacial and craniofacial surgeries. Additionally, four successful medical missions and a total of 575 surgeries were completed through the said missions in West Bengal and Andhra Pradesh.

Durgapur centre started in 2018–2019 in partnership with Operation Smile USA. A total of five missions in West Bengal, Andhra Pradesh, and Chhattisgarh were done, and 558 surgeries were completed through the missions, this very year.

A total of five missions were done in Karnataka, Odisha, West Bengal, Andhra Pradesh, and Chhattisgarh and 633 surgeries done through the missions in 2019–2020.

2021–2022 saw the establishment of two spoke centres in Siliguri and Hazaribagh, in partnership with Operation Smile USA. One medical mission was done in Vijayawada and 68 surgeries were performed through the mission the same year. Sachin Tendulkar Foundation, and corporates like HDFC ERGO, and Divgi commenced funding of cleft, maxillofacial, and craniofacial surgeries too. Furthermore, COVID-19 support activities continued with distribution of food supplies and 100 oxygen concentrators.

The foundation receives principal funding from its partnership with Operation smile. The secondary funding agencies include Allcargo Logistics Ltd., Being Human Foundation, Chandaria Foundation, Compuage Infocom Ltd., Glaxo Smith Kline, Great Eastern Shipping Corporation, Gufic Biosciences Ltd., H T Parekh Foundation, HDFC Credila Financial Services Ltd., HDFC Ergo General Insurance Company Ltd., Link Intime India Pvt Ltd., Natco Pharma Ltd., Neogen Chemicals Ltd., ORACLE, Rajratan Global Wire Ltd., Rakesh Jhunjhunwala Foundation, Sachin Tendulkar Foundation, TCFC Finance Ltd., TIH Investment Management Pvt Ltd., TTK Prestige, Ucal Fuel Systems Ltd., and Ushdev International Ltd.

The success and continued growth of the foundation are attributed not only to Dr. Krishna Shama Rao but also to the remarkable contributions of Dr. Chetana Kumar (MDS Craniofacial Surgeon and Co-founder INGA Health Foundation), Dr. Rolson Sandeep Amanna (MDS, FCFS, Fellowship AOCMF, Fellowship ICOI and Consultant, INGA Health Foundation Bangalore), Dr. Tarun Jain (MDS, Associate of the Faculty of Surgical Trainers, Fellowship in Craniofacial Surgery and Consultant, INGA Health Foundation Bangalore), and Dr. Md Shakeel Sheikh (MDS, Fellowship in Cleft and Craniofacial Surgery), who play key roles in the centre's operations.

Present Scenario of the Centre The centre is headed by two distinguished craniofacial surgeons, Dr. Krishna Shama Rao and Dr. Chetana Kumar, who lead a team of highly devoted doctors, surgeons, clinicians, and support staff. This team includes

Dr. Krishna Shama Rao, Dr. Chetana Kumar, Dr. Rolson Sandeep Amanna, Dr. Tarun Jain, Dr. Lohitha Kurupati Krishna, Dr. Centina Rose John who are all craniofacial surgeons along with Dr. Aparajita, an orthodontist, Dr. Raghavendra, a dentist and Dr. Aleena, a Speech Therapist. The support staff includes Anitha B G, Niroopa, Gaganashree Y J, and Prasanth Kumar.

Over the past few years, the centre has successfully operated numerous cases, catering to various craniofacial conditions. The centre has performed a total of 9974 surgeries since 2015 including cleft, orthognathic, maxillofacial, and craniofacial surgeries and the number of surgeries performed each year have steadily been increasing.

The centre has been offering a comprehensive range of surgical, rehabilitation and diagnostic services since 2006 to address craniofacial conditions. The surgical services include lip surgery, palate surgery, alveolar bone grafting, fistula closure, palate lengthening, VPI correction, orthognathic surgery, cleft rhinoplasty, distraction osteogenesis, craniofacial surgery, maxillofacial surgery, and surgery for vascular malformations of the head and neck. Rehabilitation services include speech therapy, audiometry, orthodontics, nasoalveolar moulding, general dentistry, nutritionist, psychologist, counsellor, and ENT services (grommet). Diagnostic services being provided at the centre include dental radiography, computed tomography, 2D echocardiography, nasoendoscopy, and videofluoroscopy.

17.1 Workflow

The workflow system at the centre begins with the identification of patients from villages or taluks by community healthcare workers, field workers, or through camps. Government doctors share the patient information with the centre, and the patients are scheduled for a visit. The patients then undergo clinical assessments by various specialists, including dentists, orthodontists, medical doctors, surgeons, and other team members. Once the necessary clearances for surgery are obtained, a surgical plan and date are determined. The centre schedules follow-up appointments post-surgery.

Challenges faced by the centre: One of the major issues faced by the centre is a lack of information about craniofacial malformations in the community and villages. While significant success has been made in raising awareness of cleft defects, the same cannot be said for more complex craniofacial deformities. This lack of understanding has resulted in a delay or even failure to discover certain malformations for timely interventions. Individuals and communities must recognise and comprehend the intricacies of craniofacial abnormalities since early intervention is critical to providing effective treatment and increasing patients' quality of life. Addressing this issue would necessitate coordinated efforts to raise awareness, educate communities, and improve public understanding of craniofacial abnormalities.

17.2 Clinical Protocol

The preferred surgical techniques at this centre include Modified Millards Rotation Advancement Cheiloplasty, Bardach and Salyer Technique, and Von-Langenbeck technique for Primary Palatoplasty and Buccal Myomucosal Flap for speech corrective surgery.

On an average, a patient needs to be admitted for about 3–4 days for primary surgeries. Suture removal is typically done after 10 days in a lip surgery.

Follow-up system at the centre requires calling the patients to the OPD or ER if they experience any fresh symptoms. Follow-ups are also arranged by Taluk/Government doctors through online mode (preferably telephonic call or Whatsapp App) as per their need and urgency.

The centre provides various support services to the patients their caregivers including accommodation, transport allowance, and food services. The patients are also provided with facilities such as PICU care, Neuro ICU care, nursing care, and consultation by a team of doctors consisting of paediatrician, anaesthetist, and surgeons. Rehabilitation services are also provided at the centre for patients.

17.3 Community Outreach

This centre is committed to providing services throughout the country, with a focus on patients within the state (90%). Referrals from primary health care centres, Cleft camps, Centre popularity (word of mouth), and Field workers help the centre reach needy patients. The foundation also has collaborations with government agencies and the National Health Mission in all respective states which help the centre broaden its reach.

17.4 Academic and Research Activities

The centre offers fellowships in cleft surgery. Some of the previous fellows include Dr. Suhas Prabhakar (Head and neck Surgeon), Dr. Tarun Jain (consultant at the Centre), Dr. Manu (consultant), Dr. Ahlem Ahamed (consultant), Dr. Hemanth Reddy (consultant), Dr. Nehal Patel (consultant), Dr. Parit (consultant), Dr. Harsha Vinay Karthik D (consultant), and Dr. Priyanka Detla among others.

This centre holds the distinction of being the only centre in India which treats all forms of craniofacial anomalies of head including craniosynostosis, hypertelorism, vascular malformations, hemifacial microsomia, Treacher Collins Syndrome, and other syndromic and non-syndromic deformities, along with the management of cleft lip and palate.

17.5 Future Direction

INGA Health intends to setup dedicated multidisciplinary centres across India over the next 5 years and train surgeons and allied professionals in line with the highest international standards. With 9000 craniofacial deformities born every year in India, the foundation envisages at least 25–30 dedicated centres across India providing state of the art care within the coming decade.

The incidence and prevalence of cleft lip and palate, and craniofacial anomalies have not changed despite having many cleft centres in India. There is a lack of experts and centres providing surgical management and comprehensive care for complex anomalies. More surgeons need to be trained for the management of cleft deformities and complex craniofacial anomalies, so as to establish centres with complete craniofacial management for those who in need.

Future centres must not only focus on providing multidisciplinary care, but also should be able to manage more complex cases. The centres must strive to enlarge their team with specialists such as interventional radiologists and neurosurgeons, to work hand-in-hand in order to deliver comprehensive care and management for craniofacial anomalies as opposed to only cleft lip and palate anomalies.

Issues such as the lack of comprehensive care in the management of craniofacial anomalies (involving skull, orbit and other vital areas), lack of awareness in the community level, as well as within the medical professionals, funding difficulties in the management of complex craniofacial deformities and lack of nutritional and psychological support need to be addressed for the successful management of cleft care.

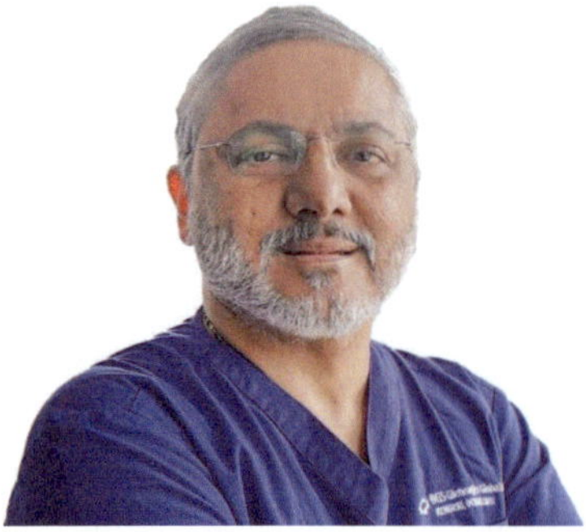

Dr. Krishna Shama Rao (Craniofacial Surgeon)

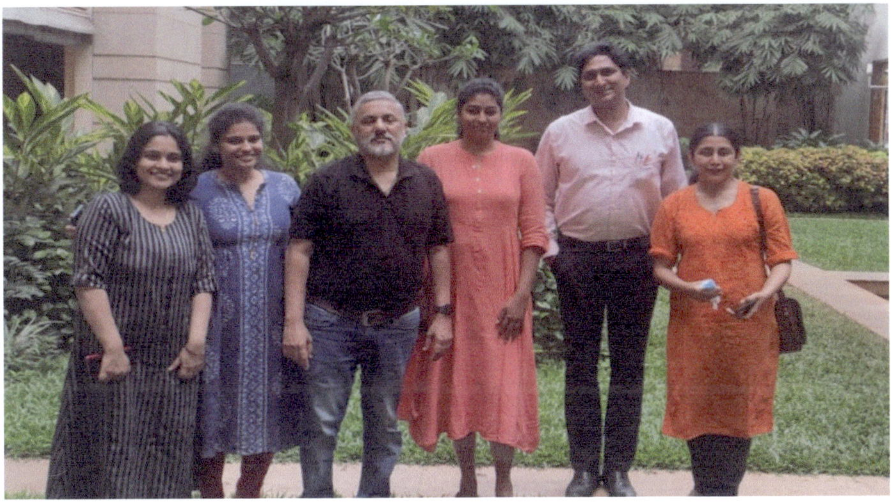

INGA Health Team. (From left to right—Dr. Centina Rose John, Dr. Lohitha Kurupati Krishna, Dr. Krishna Shama Rao, Dr. Priyanka Dedla, Dr. Rolson Sandeep, Dr. Chetana Kumar)

Chapter 18
Centre for Craniofacial Anomalies, Mangalore, Karnataka

Deborah Sybil, Hari Kishore Bhat, Akhter Husain, Shafees Koya, Faizan Ahmed Khan, and Nimalka Maria Sequeria

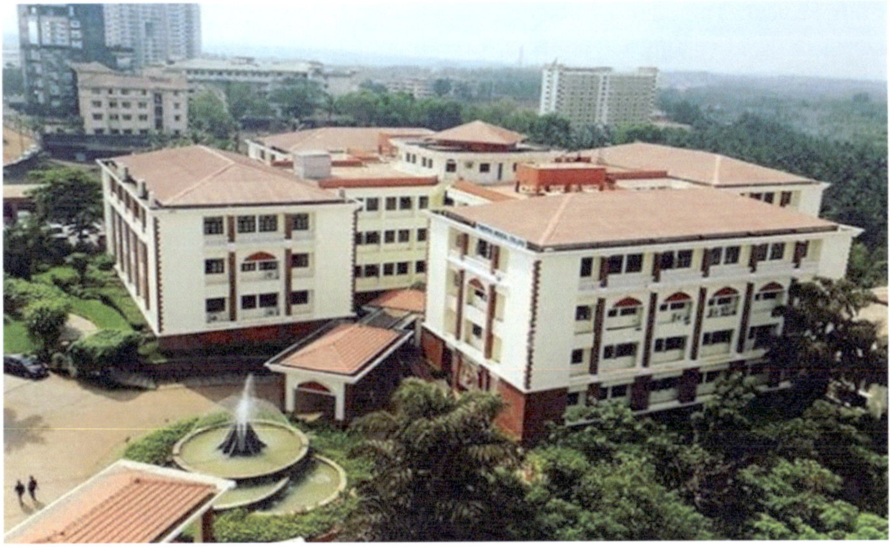

D. Sybil (✉)
Department of Oral Surgery, Faculty of Dentistry, Jamia Millia Islamia, New Delhi, India

H. K. Bhat
Centre for Craniofacial Anomalies, Yenepoya (Deemed to be University), Mangalore, India

Department of Oral & Maxillofacial Surgery, Yenepoya Dental College, Mangalore, India
e-mail: harikishore@yenepoya.edu.in

A. Husain · S. Koya · F. A. Khan
Centre for Craniofacial Anomalies, Yenepoya (Deemed to be University), Mangalore, India

Department of Orthodontics & Dentofacial Orthopaedics, Yenepoya Dental College, Mangalore, India

N. M. Sequeria
Centre for Craniofacial Anomalies, Yenepoya (Deemed to be University), Mangalore, India

P. Batra et al. (eds.), *The Cleft Care Framework in India*,
https://doi.org/10.1007/978-981-99-8968-3_18

18.1 History

The Centre for Craniofacial Anomalies was started on 17 June, 2010 by Dr. Akhter Husain (Consultant, Cleft Orthodontist) and Dr. H. Hari Kishore Bhat. The centre was infrastructurally developed in 2011 by Yenepoya (Deemed to be University) and with the introduction of speech therapy and ENT services in the year 2015–2016, the services offered got further enhanced. The centre receives funding from ABMSS (Akhila Bharatha Mahila Seva Samaja) and Yenepoya (Deemed to be University).

Present Scenario of the Centre Dr. Akhter Husain is the serving director, while Dr. H. Hari Kishore Bhat holds the position of project director, ABMSS-Yenepoya Cleft Project. The team of doctors, surgeons and clinicians include Dr. Srinivas Gosla Reddy (Visiting Craniofacial Consultant / Adjunct Professor), Dr. Shafees Koya (Consultant, Cleft Orthodontist), Dr. Faizan Ahmed Khan (Consultant, Cleft Orthodontist), Dr. Sham S Bhat (Consultant Pedodontist), Ms. Nimalka Maria Sequeria (Speech Language Pathologist & Audiologist), Dr. Mithun H K (Consultant, Paediatrician), Dr. Ravi Vaswani (Consultant, Physician), Dr.Gangadhar Somayaji (Consultant , ENT Surgeon), Dr. Deekshit R M (Consultant , ENT Surgeon), Dr. Habeeb Rehaman (Consultant Anaesthetist), Dr. Vinayak B Nayak (Consultant Anaesthetist), and Dr. Pavaman P S (Consultant Neuro surgeon).

A total of 1708 cases have been successfully operated till date at the centre. The centre has been offering a great range of surgical, rehabilitation and diagnostic services since 2011. These services include lip surgery, palate surgery, alveolar bone grafting, fistula closure, palate lengthening, VPI correction, orthognathic surgery, cleft rhinoplasty, distraction osteogenesis, speech therapy, audiometry, orthodontics, nasoalveolar molding, general dentistry, nutritionist, psychologist, counsellor, ENT services (grommet), dental radiography, computed tomography, 2D echocardiography, and nasoendoscopy.

18.2 Workflow System at the Centre

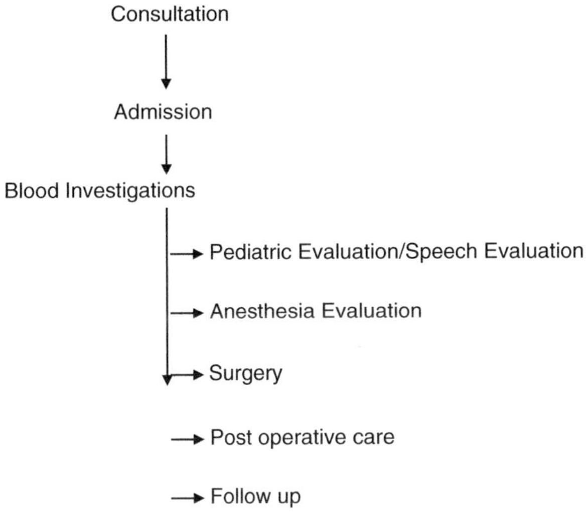

The centre experienced a marked drop in the patient flow during COVID-19.

18.3 Clinical Protocol

Afzore technique is the surgical technique for lip and palate correction preferred at the centre.

Patients undergoing primary surgeries are usually admitted for about 4–6 days depending on their individual needs. Suture removal in a lip surgery is typically done after 5–7 days of surgery and patients are communicated about their follow-up visits via phone calls. The centre also provides patient and attender accommodation, food and rehabilitation services.

18.4 Community Outreach

The centre's area of reach is within a radius of 200 km from its location (Mangalore). Referrals from primary health care centres and Centre's popularity (word of mouth) remain the two most important means of the centre's reach to needy patients. The centre has also collaborated with various government agencies and primary health centres in order to provide more and more community-based services.

18.5 Academic and Research Activities

This centre offers four fellowships in cleft in addition to carrying out researches in this domain. Two of these researches include NAMUC Study (Multi centric Clinical Trial) and a PhD on Predisposing factors of cleft.

18.6 Future Direction

The centre's future vision is centred around optimising patient flow along with providing quality comprehensive care. Centre for craniofacial anomalies believes in and thus advises rigorous training for next generation of cleft care personnel besides being empathetic in delivering comprehensive cleft care as well as developing and following a system of meticulous documentation.

The centre strongly believes in the development of comprehensive care centres with multidisciplinary approach. Despite best efforts, clinical registry for Clefts in India and consensus on treatment planning and techniques are still lacking in India which needs attention.

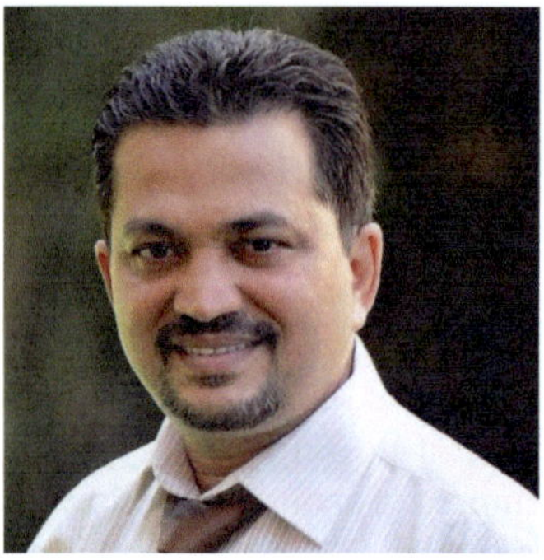

Dr. Akhter Husain (Orthodontist)

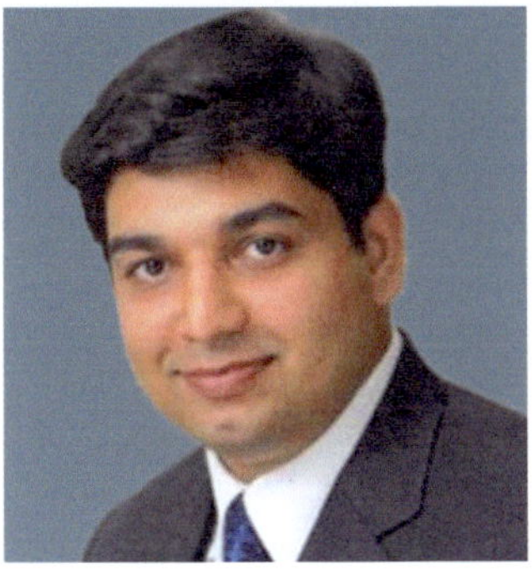

Dr. H. Hari Kishore Bhat (Oral and Maxillofacial Surgeon)

Chapter 19
The Cleft and Craniofacial Centre, Sree Balaji Medical College & Hospital and Dr Rela Institute & Medical Centre, Chennai, Tamil Nadu

Badri Thiruvenkatachari, Syed Altaf Hussain, Charanya Vijayakumar, Badri Thiruvenkatachari, and B. Subramaniyan

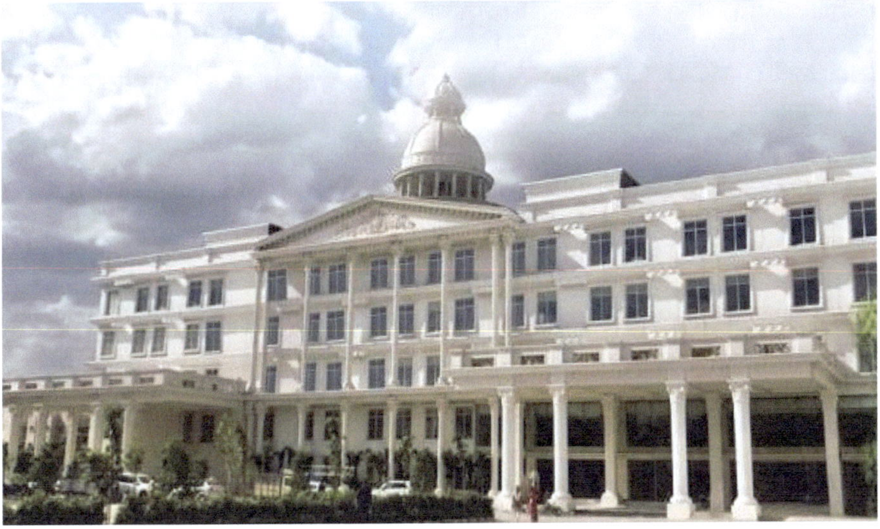

B. Thiruvenkatachari (✉) · B. Thiruvenkatachari
Research, Sree Balaji Dental College and Hospital, BIHER, Chennai, India

Orthodontics, University of Manchester, Manchester, UK

S. A. Hussain · C. Vijayakumar
Department of Plastic and Reconstructive Surgery, Sree Balaji Medical College and Hospital, The Cleft and Craniofacial Centre, Chennai, India

B. Subramaniyan
Department of Speech-Language Pathology, Sree Balaji Medical College and Hospital, The Cleft and Craniofacial Centre, Chennai, India

P. Batra et al. (eds.), *The Cleft Care Framework in India*,
https://doi.org/10.1007/978-981-99-8968-3_19

History of the Centre The Cleft and Craniofacial Centre, Sree Balaji Medical College & Hospital and Dr. Rela Institute was established on 1 June, 2022 owing success to the pioneer Dr. Syed Altaf Hussain as well as the team of dedicated staff whose roles cannot be overlooked including Dr. Charanya Vijayakumar, Dr. Badri Thiruvenkatachari, and Dr. S. Bhuminathan, among others. The centre's principal and secondary funding agencies include Sree Balaji Medical College and Hospital, Dr. Rela Institute and Medical Centre, Smile Train, Ekam Foundation, and Vijay Amritraj Foundation.

Present Scenario of the Centre Dr. Syed Altaf Hussain, a plastic surgeon, is the Centre Head who leads the team of highly skilled doctors, surgeons, clinicians, and support staff. The team comprises of Dr. Charanya Vijayakumar (Oral and Maxillofacial surgeon), Dr. Badri Thiruvenkatachari (Lead Orthodontist), Dr. Manoj Pratap C (Orthodontist), Dr. Subhiksha (Orthodontist), Dr. Karthika Nambiar (Orthodontist), Dr. Vivekandandan (ENT surgeon), Dr. Subramaniyan B (Lead Speech and Language Pathologist), Ms. Swetha Sridhar (Speech and Language Pathologist), Ms. Deepalakshmi Sriram (Paediatric and Neonatal Nutritionist), Mr. Jayakumar (Patient Facilitator), Ms. Sahana C (Senior Executive Admin and Accounts), Ms Gomathi, Ms Rajakumari, Dis Sumi and Ms Anu.

The centre has been offering a wide range of surgical and rehabilitation services since July 1, 2022 along with nasoendoscopy for diagnostic purpose. The surgical services currently being offered at the centre include lip surgery, palate surgery, alveolar bone grafting, fistula closure, palate lengthening, VPI correction, orthognathic surgery, cleft rhinoplasty, and distraction osteogenesis and the rehabilitation services include speech therapy, orthodontics, nasoalveolar moulding, general dentist, nutritionist and ENT services (Grommet).

Clinical Protocol The centre follows an organised 3-day schedule for surgery wherein the patient is assessed for surgical fitness along with preoperative investigations and hence admission if found fit for surgery on the first day. Surgery is then performed on day 2 and the third day comprises of immediate post-operative care, counselling on care of surgical site, feeding and medication advice and finally discharge if the patient needs no additional care.

Suture removal in case of lip surgery is done on post-operative day 5 to allow optimal healing.

Follow-up system at the centre: The centre has an extensive follow-up system in place. Lip operated patients are reviewed on post-operative day 5 for suture removal, while palate operated patients are reviewed 2 weeks post-discharge. All patients who receive surgical interventions are regularly followed up with the team over phone calls to make sure they are free from post-operative complications. Additionally, the patients who undergo lip surgeries are counselled for scar massage after suture removal.

Community Outreach The centre actively participates in various community services and collaborates with government agencies and primary health centres for support. Dr. Subramaniyan B, Professor and consultant Speech Language Pathologist had a meeting with Dr.Balasubramanian, Director—RUWSEC (Rural Women's Social Education Centre), Thirukazhukundram to explore the possible collaboration for outreach programmes on September 30, 2022. An online meeting was also conducted with Ms. Alphina Jose Thambi - Vice President, BWDA (Bullock-cart Workers Development Association), Villupuram to initiate awareness programmes for sensitising grass root level workers about cleft lip and palate. Dr. Subramaniyan B, Professor and consultant Speech Language Pathologist was interviewed about treatment for Cleft Lip and Palate by BWDA community radio channel based in Villupuram. These programmes are a testament to centre's dedication towards raising awareness about cleft care.

Academic and Research Activities Sree Balaji Dental College and Hospital Cleft and Craniofacial department headed by Dr. Badri Thiruvenkatachari has been awarded a research grant of 4.68 Crores to improve the quality of life and reduce the treatment burden for patients with cleft lip and palate. This is the largest grant to be awarded to any dental institution in the country. The grant comes from Department of Biotechnology, India and Wellcome Trust, UK (India Alliance) to look into the effectiveness of a nasoalveolar moulding (NAM) treatment for babies born with cleft lip and palate.

The Cleft and Craniofacial Centre, Sree Balaji Medical College & Hospital and Dr. Rela Institute has a short yet phenomenal history of providing holistic care to cleft lip and palate patients. With a devoted team, cutting edge facilities, dedication to research and community outreach, the centre strives to make a difference in the lives of patients with cleft deformities.

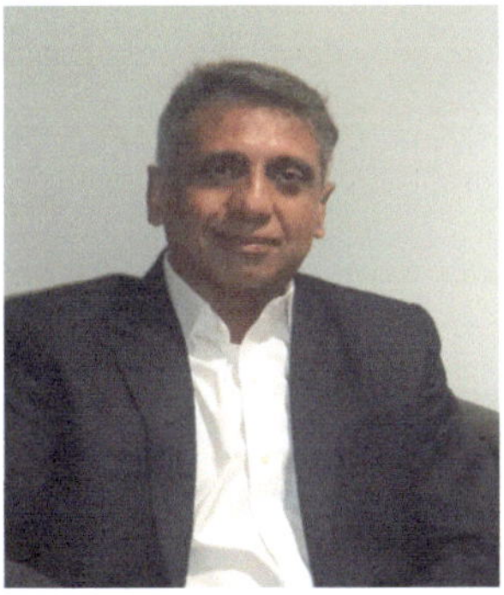

Dr. Syed Altaf Hussain (Plastic Surgeon)

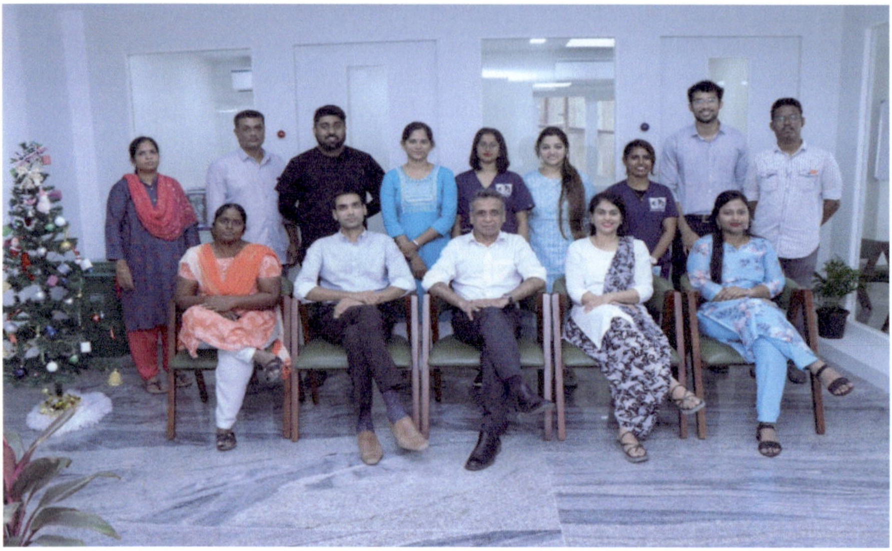

The Cleft care team. *Standing from left to right:* **Gomathy sis – Speech, Jaya Kumar – Driver, Dr. Manoj Prathap – Research Fellow, Dr. Subiksha – Research Fellow, Dr. Deepa – Nutritionist, Dr. Kartika – Research Fellow, Swetha – Speech Pathologist, Yadhu – Physician Assistant, Samuel – Coordinator,** *Sitting from right to left:* **Sahana – Administrator, Dr. Charanya – OMFS – SMILE TRAIN Surgeon, Dr. Syed Altaff Hussain – HOD – PLASTIC SURGEON, Dr. Badri Thiruvenkatachari – Orthodontic Lead, Sis Jhansi – Feeding nurse**

Chapter 20
ABMSS Comprehensive Cleft Care (CCC) Centre, Bangalore, Karnataka

Panchali Batra, Dushyant Prasad, and B. S. Jayanth

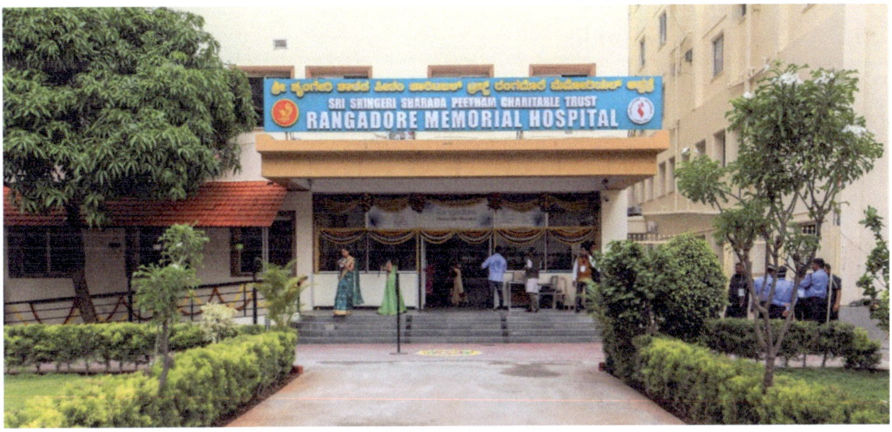

20.1 History

The ABMSS Comprehensive Cleft Care (CCC) Centre, located at Bangalore Rangadore Memorial Hospital in Bangalore, started in June 2018.

The centre got wings to take off to cater to the needs of comprehensive cleft care for the thousands of odd cleft children born each year in various districts of Karnataka. The hospital being a well-known neonatal/paediatric care hospital offered an ideal launch pad with availability of NICU/PICU and paediatric anaesthetist to safely handle all primary cleft surgeries. Understanding the importance of providing a comprehensive circle of care to cleft families, including nutrition,

P. Batra (✉)
Department of Orthodontics, Faculty of Dentistry, Jamia Millia Islamia, New Delhi, India
e-mail: p.batra@jmi.ac.in

D. Prasad · B. S. Jayanth
Rangadore Memorial Hospital, Bengaluru, Karnataka, India
e-mail: jayanth.b.s@spaltkinder.org

P. Batra et al. (eds.), *The Cleft Care Framework in India*,
https://doi.org/10.1007/978-981-99-8968-3_20

NAM, medical support, speech services, ENT treatments and surgeries, dental treatment, orthodontic treatment, counselling, and all stages of cleft surgeries until the child is integrated into society as an adult, the centre was established as a CCC since the very beginning. The centre successfully treated over a hundred patients in its first year of service, and the number of families getting services has grown remarkably over time, with the centre now assisting more than 400 families annually. Despite the challenges posed by the COVID-19 pandemic, the centre has treated over 1157 cleft children.

20.2 Present Scenario

Dr. Jayanth B S has led the centre since its start, advocating for CCC services not only for Karnataka patients, but also for those from Tamil Nadu, Kerala, and Andhra Pradesh, resulting in a multiplier effect for the centre's impact.

Under Dr. Jayanth's guidance, a dedicated CCC team was formed, consisting of cleft fellows Dr. Prithvi, Dr. Shobha Hegde, Dr. Shreya BM, and other professionals including Dr. Kavya (Paediatric Anaesthesist), Dr. Amuktha (Anaesthesist), Dr. Gupta (Anaesthesist), Dr. Guruprasad (PICU), Dr. Prasad (NICU), Dr. Nidhi S (PICU), Dr. Subramanya Rao (ENT), Dr. Babu (ENT), Dr. Sandhya (ENT), Dr. Gautam (orthodontist), Dr. Prajwal (orthodontist), Dr. Preethi Menon (prosthodontist), Dr. Shruthi (Dentist), Dr. Ankitha (Dentist), and speech therapists Mrs. Srividya, Ms. Fathima, and Ms. Shifali along with the centre coordinator, Mr. Sagar and the field animator, Mr. Swamy to ensure the smooth functioning of this centre.

The primary funding agency is ABMSS which is the second largest cleft NGO in the country.

The centre has conducted approximately 971 surgeries to date. The centre supports the treatment of underprivileged children born with cleft lip and palate deformities with free surgery and comprehensive cleft care which includes NAM, nutrition, speech therapy, orthodontics, ENT (to prevent hearing loss and eventual learning disability in school), dentistry, transportation, food and post-operative medicines, and follow-up care appropriate to the age and need of each case. To achieve this Circle of Care, every child is closely monitored using a strong database and a unique Cleft Passport mechanism to make sure that their growth is documented from birth until they become integrated members of society as near normal adults. The centre not only supports primary surgeries but also secondary procedures as the child grows, including 6–7 surgical (Distraction osteogenesis included) and 5 ancillary care services, without any age restrictions.

The centre also supports in house 2D echo, CT scans, ultrasound scans, videolaryngoscopy, nasal endoscopy, and entire range of blood investigations to support the burden of congenital care.

20.3 Workflow

The centre gets its patients through outreach work across the state of Karnataka and its neighbouring states for which it has an exclusive field animator who is in field work all through the year. Camps are also frequently organised with public offices of the Govt. of Karnataka through Health and Education department to advocate CCC and functional rehabilitation. A good proportion of cases do walk in through professional referral and word of mouth. Patients are counselled at the centre based on the stage and diagnosis they present with. After that, they are entered into the database and given a Cleft Passport with a unique number. They then undergo the necessary workup and are referred to appropriate CCC services. Due to the presence of multiple professionals in each CCC team, most patients benefit from maximal intervention during a single visit, minimising downtime for their families. ABMSS is currently the sole funding source for the centre.

The major headwinds are the fragile ecosystem of social work, including travel logistics for families, limited availability of beds and wards for accompanying family members, challenges from local administration who fail to understand the nature of work in rural areas, increasing logistics costs, demand for pay parity within the hospital and the team, limited resources for special investigations of syndromic cases, and difficulties in monitoring school children, especially after their return to school following the pandemic.

The centre mainly prefers Fischers anatomic subunit technique for Cleft lip repair, Bardach's 2 flap with Buccal fat pad for the raw area coverage in complete cleft palate, Wardill-Kilner technique or Traditional Vonlagenback's technique for incomplete cleft palate and Furlows for Submucous cleft palate. The average stay for most patients is 3 days in the hospital with most of them coming back on Day 8 for a checkup along with suture removal.

20.4 Clinical Protocol

The centre's comprehensive cleft care programme offers an organised treatment plan for children from the time they are born until they have their primary lip surgery done. Initially, the child visits the centre on weekly basis for nasoalveolar moulding. After the lip closure, bimonthly checkups are scheduled until the palate is repaired. Once the palate is repaired, the child has annual visits for speech evaluation and stimulation until therapy begins at the age of 3.5 years. These appointments also involve ENT and dental check-ups. As the child grows, procedures such as speech improvement surgery, lip revision, or fistula repair may be required, which are done between the ages of 4 and 6 years based on appropriate indications. Then the child begins mixed dentition orthodontics to expand the arch or initiate growth modifying therapy before bone grafting, which is usually done between 9 and 11 years of age based on the stage of canine eruption. Annual visits continue to monitor dental and ENT health, speech progress, and overall growth during this entire period. They undergo presurgical orthodontics thereafter and are ready for jaw advancement and final rhinoplasty following their adolescence growth cessation.

Almost all surgical and CCC services are free along with transportation and food support for the patients and their attendants during each visit.

20.5 Community Outreach

The centre's reach extends across the entire state of Karnataka and bordering districts of Andhra Pradesh, Tamil Nadu, and Kerala. Patients reach here for treatment through camps organised by the field animator, professional referrals, word of mouth, and collaborations with government programmes like RBSK and SSK.

20.6 Academic and Research Activities

Centre has been supporting Fellowship post pandemic in CCC only and hence currently one fellow has completed the programme.

20.7 Future Direction

In the future, the centre aims to fill the gaps in comprehensive cleft care for children in Karnataka and contribute to training future doctors in the philosophy of CCC, emphasising the importance of holistic treatment and not just surgery which would defeat the very purpose of treating such children by cosmetically concealing their faces.

The next generation of care providers need to take this up as service and not as a source of earning as this is a long-drawn love affair with cleft children; investing their time, enthusiasm, skills and efforts over a lifetime to achieve something tangible not just for the cleft community but for their own professional satisfaction.

Cleft care in India lacks standardisation of cleft infrastructure, a cleft registry at state level, proper awareness and advocacy for CCC, adequate funding to support the full scope of CCC for every child including parental support programmes and last but not the least a centralised data management of the health records of these cleft cases transcending the boundaries of cleft care providers.

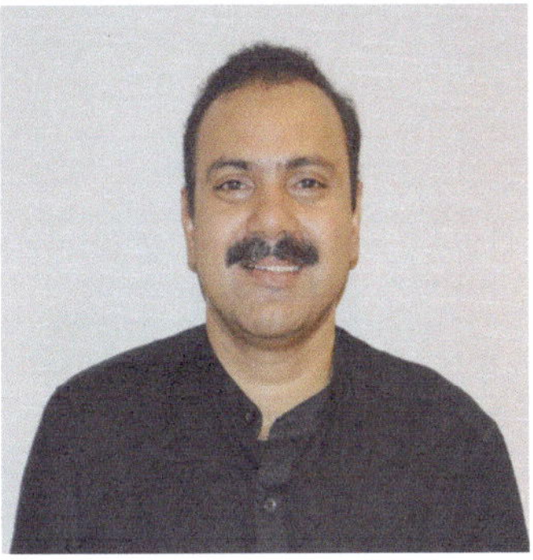

Dr. Jayanth B S (Oral and Maxillofacial Surgeons)

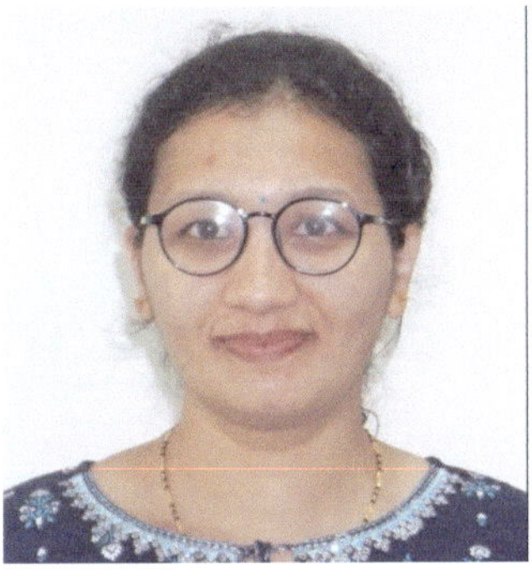

Dr. Shobha (Oral and Maxillofacial Surgeons)

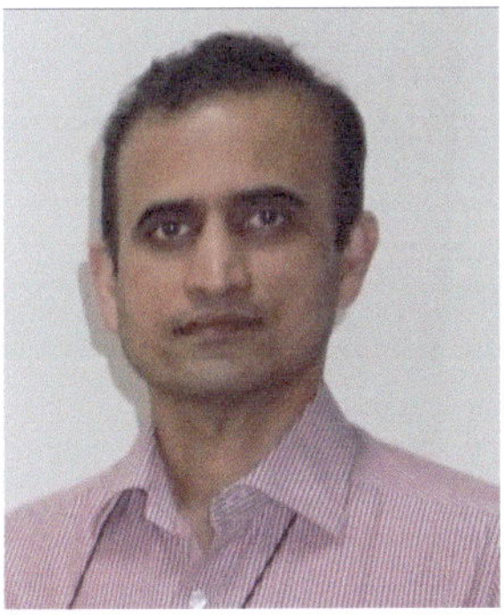

Dr. Subramanya Rao (ENT specialist)

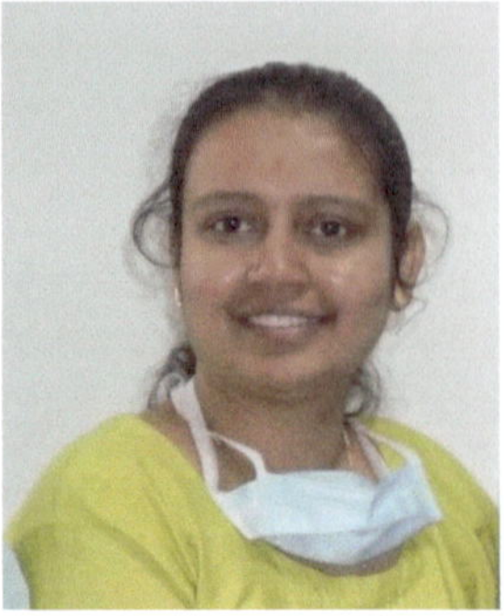

Dr. Ankita (Dentist)

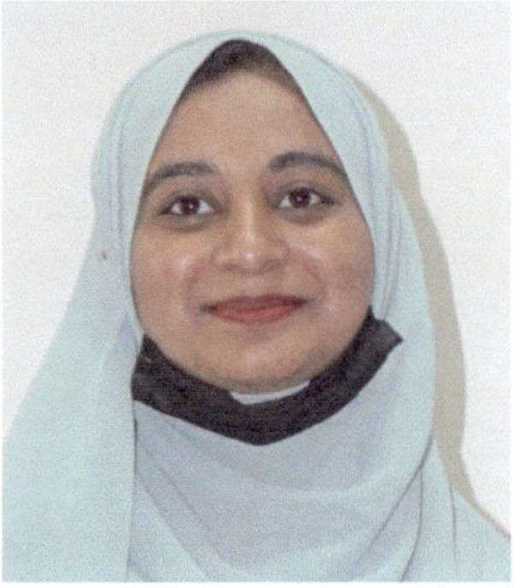

Dr. Fathima (Speech Therapist)

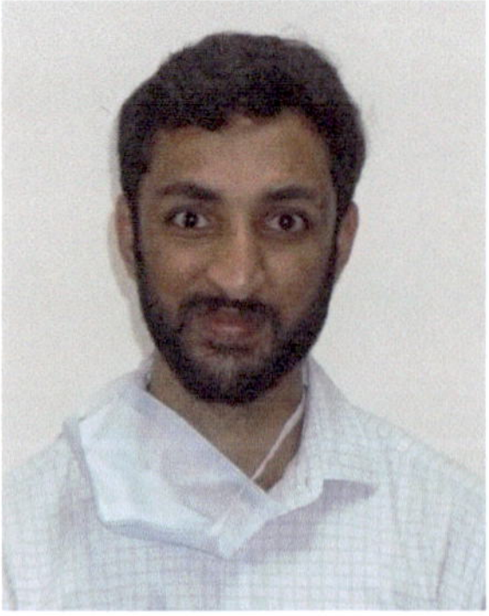

Sagar (Centre Coordinator)

Chapter 21
ABMSS Comprehensive Cleft Care (CCC) Centre, Hyderabad, Telangana

Panchali Batra, Dushyant Prasad, and Vijay Kumar

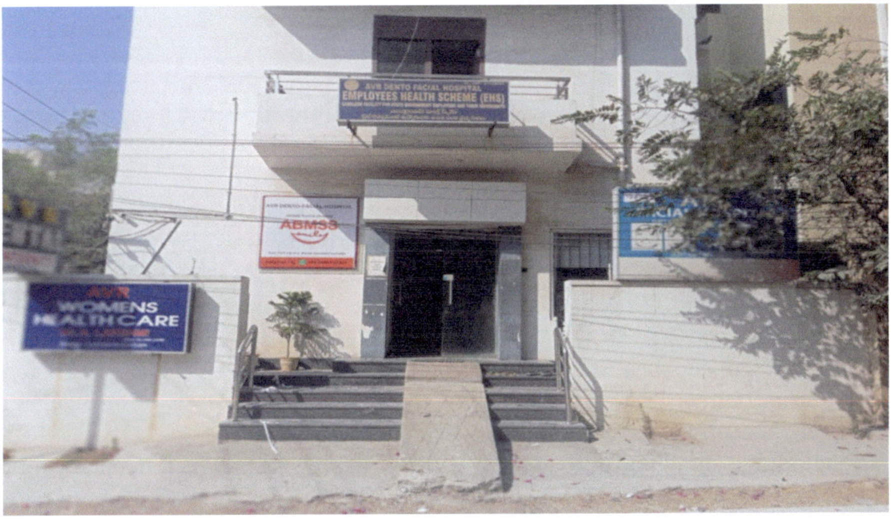

21.1 History and Milestones

ABMSS Comprehensive Cleft Care (CCC) Centre, located at AVR Dental Facial Hospital in Hyderabad, is a pioneering centre that started its operations in April 2015. Initially established as a cleft care centre, it has gradually evolved into a comprehensive cleft care facility. The centre has been a blessing for thousands of children born with cleft lip and palate deformities, who previously lacked access to

P. Batra (✉)
Department of Orthodontics, Faculty of Dentistry, Jamia Millia Islamia, New Delhi, India
e-mail: p.batra@jmi.ac.in

D. Prasad · V. Kumar
AVR Hospital, Hyderabad, Telangana, India
e-mail: dushyant.prasad@abmss.in

P. Batra et al. (eds.), *The Cleft Care Framework in India*,
https://doi.org/10.1007/978-981-99-8968-3_21

quality services in the state. Equipped with paediatric care specialized for cleft conditions, the centre recognized the need to provide a comprehensive circle of care for these children. This circle of care includes nutrition support, NAM, medical assistance, speech services, ENT care (including surgeries), dental treatment, orthodontic treatment, counselling, and all stages of cleft surgeries until the child is integrated into society as an adult. In response to the unmet need for comprehensive cleft care, the centre was transformed into a CCC in 2019. In its first year as a CCC, the centre served over a hundred patients, and since then, the number has gradually increased, currently providing services to more than 450 families annually. Over the years, the centre has performed surgeries on 2000 cleft children from the states of Telangana and Andhra Pradesh.

21.2 Present Scenario

The success of the ABMSS CCC Centre can be attributed to the dedicated efforts of several individuals. Dr. Dushyant Prasad, Dr. Jayanth B S, Dr. Uday, and Md. Afroz has played major roles in the establishment and advocacy of the CCC, along with Dr. A. Vijay Kumar. The centre is staffed by trained professionals such as Dr. Uday Kumar (Anaesthesia), Dr. Shashi (Paediatrician), Dr. Sreedevi (Cardiologist), Srilatha (Head Nursing Staff), and Md. Afroz (Animator Incharge), and Cleft Coordinator Athiya Khatoon. The centre also collaborates with Dr. Yogander for ENT care and surgery and Akrithi for speech evaluation.

The primary funding for the centre comes from ABMSS, which happens to be the second largest cleft NGO in the country. Since its inception, the centre has performed approximately 2000 surgeries. The centre focuses not only on primary surgeries but also provides support for secondary procedures as the child grows, including various bony procedures like distraction osteogenesis. This comprehensive approach ensures that the child receives continuous care throughout their growth and development until adulthood, without any age restrictions. The centre covers the costs of surgeries, transportation, food, post-operative medicines, and follow-up care, ensuring that underprivileged children with cleft deformities receive the necessary treatment free of charge. To ensure effective monitoring and follow-up, each child is tracked from birth through a robust database and cleft passport mechanism, ensuring their progress is monitored regularly until they are integrated into society as near-normal adults. The ABMSS CCC Centre is committed to providing comprehensive care to cleft-affected children, supporting them not just in primary surgeries but also in secondary procedures and ancillary care services.

The centre also supports in-house 2D ECHO, CT scans, ultrasound scans, videolaryngoscopy, nasal endoscopy, and the entire range of blood investigations to support the burden of congenital care.

21.3 Workflow

The centre operates with an average of 25 surgeries per month, reaching out to patients through extensive outreach work across the states of Telangana and Andhra Pradesh. To facilitate this, the centre has a dedicated Field Animator who conducts fieldwork throughout the year. Additionally, the centre collaborates with public offices of the Government of Telangana, particularly the Health and Education departments, to organize camps and promote comprehensive cleft care and functional rehabilitation. Many patients are also referred to the Centre by professionals and through word of mouth, while social media platforms such as Facebook and WhatsApp also play a role in patient referrals.

Upon arrival at the Centre, patients undergo counselling for comprehensive cleft care based on their specific stage of treatment and diagnosis. They are then registered into the database and provided with a Cleft Passport that bears a unique identification number. Following registration, patients proceed through the work-up process and are referred to the Comprehensive Cleft Care (CCC) team. One advantage of the Centre is that most patients can receive maximum intervention during a single visit, as each CCC team consists of multiple professionals, thereby minimizing downtime for the families.

However, the centre faces several challenges in its workflow. One significant challenge is the fragile ecosystem of social work, including logistical issues related to travel for the families, as they expect the Centre to arrange transportation from pick-up to drop-off. Furthermore, there is a lack of beds and wards for patient families who wish to accompany their children during treatment. The centre also encounters challenges from local administration officials who may not fully comprehend the nature of their work in rural areas. Additionally, the logistics and cost involved in recruiting patients, which often involve middlemen, pose ongoing challenges. The centre also receives regular demands from the hospital and other team members to ensure pay parity. Special investigations for syndromic children can be challenging due to limited resources, and there are difficulties in following up with school children, especially after their return to school following the pandemic.

To support all these activities, the centre relies heavily on funding from ABMSS. This funding helps cover the costs associated with patient care, counselling, surgeries, logistics, and other essential aspects of the Centre's operations.

The centre mainly does Modified Millard and Afroz'e Technique for Cleft lip repair, whereas Veau-Wardill-Kilner, Von Langenback's V-Y Pushback technique for incomplete cleft palate and a Furlows for Submucous cleft palate. The average stay for most patients is 2 days in the hospital with most of them coming back on Days 8–10 for a check-up along with suture removal. The centre also encourages the patient to come for an annual check-up to see the progress of the surgery.

21.4 Clinical Protocol

The Cleft Care Center (CCC) follows a comprehensive care pathway for children from inception until primary lip surgery and beyond. Initially, the child visits the centre for NAM weekly. After lip closure, the visits are scheduled bimonthly until the palate is repaired. Once the palate repair is completed, the child undergoes annual visits for speech assessment and stimulation until therapy begins at 3.5 years of age. These visits also include ENT and dental check-ups. Between the ages of 4 and 6, the patients may undergo speech improvement surgery, lip revision, or fistula repair based on the appropriate indications. From the age of 9–11, they start mixed dentition orthodontics to expand the arch or initiate growth-modifying therapy before the bone grafting, considering the stage of canine eruption. Throughout the annual visits, the centre monitors the dental and ENT health, speech progress, and growth of the children. Presurgical orthodontics are performed, followed by jaw advancement and final rhinoplasty after the cessation of adolescent growth.

The centre provides almost all surgical and CCC services for free, including transportation and food support for both the patient and their family during each visit.

21.5 Community Outreach

The centre covers the entire state of Telangana and the bordering districts of Andhra Pradesh. Patients are brought in through camps organized by field animators, professional referrals, word of mouth, and government tie-ups through programmes like RBSK (Rashtriya Bal Swasthta Karyakram) and SSA (Sarva Shiksha Abhiyan).

21.6 Academic and Research Activities

Since 2017, the centre has been supporting a fellowship programme, providing training in cleft and craniofacial surgeries. This ensures the continuous development of skilled care providers in the field. However, there is a need for further expansion as the centre plans to start four outreach programmes about 200 km away to provide additional facilities to children in the state.

21.7 Future Direction

The next generation of care providers must possess passion, compassion, and empathy towards the cleft society. They should invest their time, enthusiasm, skills, and efforts over a lifetime to achieve tangible results, not just for the cleft community but also for their professional satisfaction.

In India, cleft care lacks standardization of infrastructure, a cleft registry at the state level, proper awareness and advocacy for CCC, and adequate funding to support the full scope of CCC for every child, including parental support programmes. Moreover, there is a need for proper surgical training and orientation towards CCC in the country.

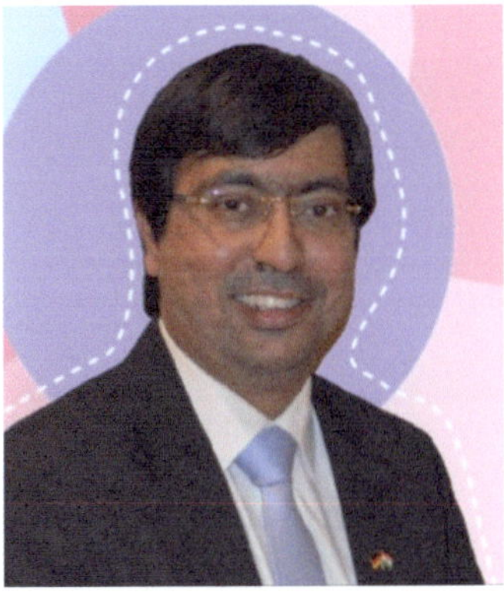

Dr. Dushyant Prasa (Founder)

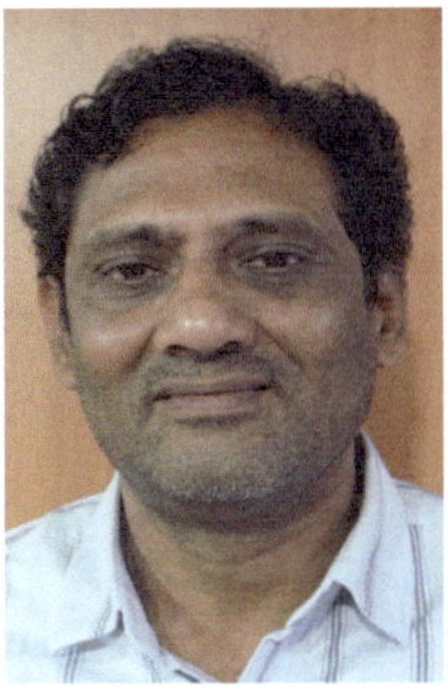

Dr. Vijay Kumar (Maxillofacial Surgeon)

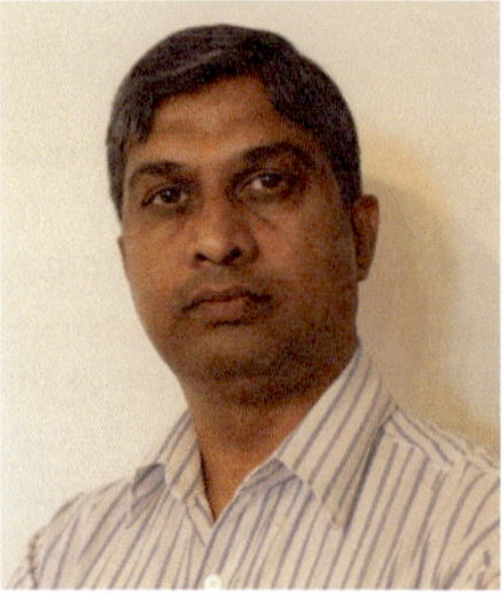

Dr. Uday Kiran (Anesthesiologist)

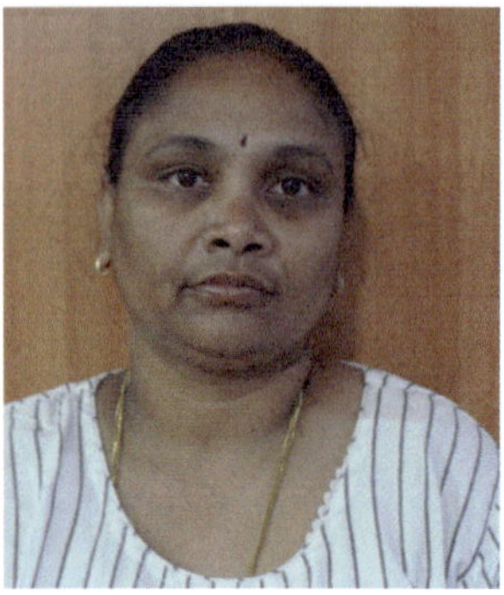

Dr. Keerthi (Dentist)

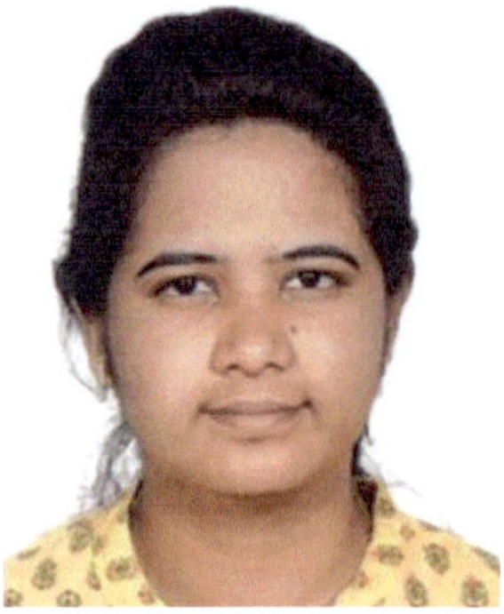

Dr. Nikita Reddy (Orthodontist)

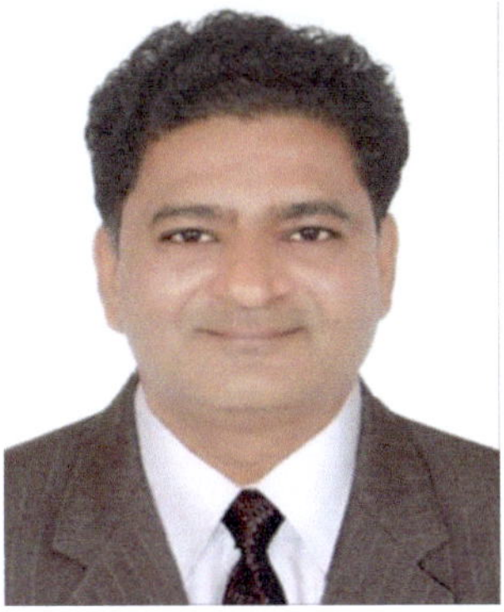

Dr. Yougender (ENT Specialist)

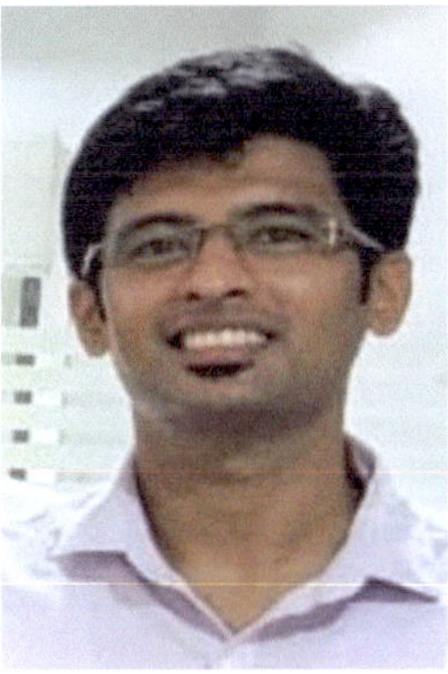

Dr. Harish (Assisting doctor)

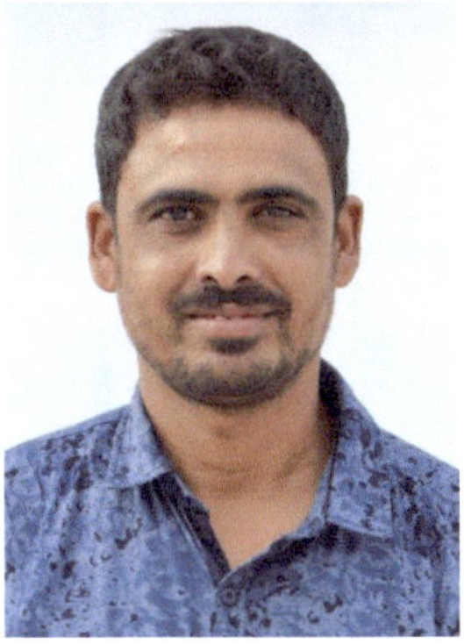

Afroz Taj (Centre coordinator)

Part VII
Our Recommendations and Way Forward: The CCIS Study

Chapter 22
Future Recommendations for Enhancing Cleft Care

Badri Thiruvenkatachari, Deborah Sybil, Krishnamurthy Bonanthaya, and Panchali Batra

Over the years, significant progress has been made in cleft care in India, with awareness campaigns, better access and an increase in financial resources, contributing to improved outcomes. However, there is still ample room for enhancement. This section delves into the ways in which cleft care in India can be further improved to ensure comprehensive and accessible treatment for all affected individuals.

22.1 Timely Diagnosis

One of the key aspects of enhancing cleft care is timely diagnosis and early intervention. By promoting awareness among expectant mothers and healthcare providers, early diagnosis of cleft conditions can be facilitated. Although there is not much data available on prenatal diagnosis of cleft in India, we feel there is only a very small percentage of mothers are being diagnosed prenatally. There is a lack of coordination between radiologists, midwives, cleft teams, and parents to provide better diagnosis and care pathways for pregnant mothers with cleft babies. Prenatal counselling can help understand the condition and prepare for the journey ahead. Health professionals should receive training to identify cleft cases during routine examinations, enabling timely referral to specialised centres. A care pathway from diagnosis to treatment needs to be established and quality checks should be in place to make

B. Thiruvenkatachari (✉)
Dental Research, Sree Balaji Medical and Dental Colleges and Hospital, The Cleft and Craniofacial Centre, Chennai, India

D. Sybil · P. Batra
Department of Oral Surgery, Faculty of Dentistry, Jamia Millia Islamia, New Delhi, India

K. Bonanthaya
Bhagwan Mahaveer Jain Hospital, Bangalore, India

P. Batra et al. (eds.), *The Cleft Care Framework in India*,
https://doi.org/10.1007/978-981-99-8968-3_22

sure parents are being supported and cared for. The implementation of the above can be made possible by bringing together different specialist associations involved in the care and awareness promoted through the associations.

22.2 Early Intervention

Early intervention is a cornerstone of effective cleft care. Timely diagnosis and treatment during infancy can significantly improve a child's and parents' quality of life. Therefore, investing in improved diagnostic tools and training for healthcare providers is crucial. Training radiologists in visualising and identifying any potential cleft abnormalities should be taken as a priority. Additionally, there should be a clear care pathway for radiologists to refer potential cleft babies to appropriate comprehensive cleft centres so early intervention can be provided. Better coordination is required between public and private sector healthcare workers in identifying and treating cleft babies. There is still a lack of coordination between NGO-funded care and public hospitals, in some areas across India. The timely referral from public maternity departments to NGO/public-funded comprehensive cleft care centres should be improved. This can be carried out by raising awareness among public and private maternity departments and implementing appropriate policies from healthcare policymakers.

22.3 Strengthening Access to Care

While progress has been made in urban areas, rural and underserved regions often lack adequate access to cleft care services. Mobile clinics and outreach programmes can bridge this gap by bringing medical professionals and resources to these communities. Government collaboration with NGOs and private healthcare institutions can facilitate the establishment of specialised cleft care centres in remote areas, ensuring that no individual is left without proper treatment due to geographical limitations. There should be a national database on comprehensive cleft care centres, with clear information on referral pathways and access, which can be accessed by both caretakers of babies with cleft and healthcare workers.

22.4 Interdisciplinary Approach

A comprehensive approach involving a multidisciplinary team is crucial for effective cleft care. Plastic surgeons, speech therapists, orthodontists, and psychologists should work collaboratively to address the physical, speech, and psychological aspects of the condition. Regular team meetings and coordinated treatment plans can result in more holistic care and better outcomes. Healthcare policymakers should work on establishing more publicly funded comprehensive cleft care centres in rural areas. There is a serious lack of comprehensive cleft care centres providing high-quality treatment in both rural and urban areas. Healthcare policymakers should work with NGOs and other private healthcare workers in developing a workforce planning strategy to ensure that the right number of skilled and qualified healthcare professionals are available to meet the current and future needs of cleft patients and the healthcare system.

22.5 Education and Awareness

Educating communities about cleft conditions is pivotal in reducing stigma and improving acceptance. Educational campaigns can be conducted through schools, community centres, and digital platforms. Providing accurate information about available treatments, rehabilitation options, and success stories can empower families and individuals to seek appropriate care without hesitation.

22.6 Strengthening Rehabilitation Services

Rehabilitation, including speech therapy and psychosocial support, is integral to cleft care. There is a serious lack of speech pathologists and psychologists working in cleft care. Expanding the availability of speech therapists in both urban and rural areas is crucial to improving the overall quality of care in India. Although there is some access to speech in NGO-funded care, there is absolutely no access to speech in rural public-funded cleft centres. Our healthcare policymakers and politicians should team up and develop a strategy to recruit and retain speech pathologists in rural cleft centres. While there is limited access to psychologists in both private and public/NGO-funded cleft centres, support groups can help individuals cope with the emotional challenges associated with cleft conditions.

22.7 Research and Data Collection

Research plays a pivotal role in understanding the prevalence, causes, and long-term outcomes of cleft conditions. Establishing a national registry for cleft cases can help healthcare providers gather valuable data, track progress, and identify areas requiring improvement. High-quality research on a national level involving multi-centric trials is crucial in providing high-quality care for our patients. National audits should be initiated to assess and improve the quality of care. Audits help in providing a benchmark for quality and to make sure that the low-outcome quality centre has an opportunity to train and improve the quality of care. These regular audits are mandatory to maintain the quality and to keep patients safe.

22.8 Financial Support and Public–Private Partnerships

Cleft care can be financially burdensome for many families, particularly those from low-income backgrounds. Governments, NGOs, and private entities should collaborate to provide financial assistance, insurance coverage, and grants for treatment. Public–private partnerships can lead to sustainable initiatives that address the financial challenges associated with cleft care. Our healthcare policymakers, politicians, healthcare providers, and other stakeholders should work together to develop strategies for providing financial support, access, and improved quality of care.

22.9 Training and Capacity Building

A skilled workforce is essential for providing quality cleft care. Governments and institutions should invest in training programmes for healthcare professionals, ensuring that they have the necessary skills to address the diverse needs of cleft patients. Specialised cleft training programmes are required to train young clinicians to manage the complexity involved in cleft care. Government organisations should team up with private non-profitable institutions in developing comprehensive cleft training programmes. These centres can also work as a "hub" providing services and resources, while also establishing specialised "bespoke" units in limited access areas reducing patients' travel burden without compromising care quality.

In conclusion, enhancing cleft care requires a multifaceted approach that spans early diagnosis, early intervention, access to care, multidisciplinary collaboration, education, research, and financial support. By combining the efforts of governments, NGOs, healthcare institutions, and communities, we can create a more comprehensive and accessible cleft care system. Ultimately, the goal is to provide individuals born with cleft lip and palate the opportunity to lead fulfilling lives, free from the burdens of their condition.

Recommendations of Cleft Care India Study

1. Identification of statewise cleft leadership personnel, willing to develop a network and referral system for the state.
2. Identification of statewise cleft care centres where cleft treatment is being provided (including identification of infrastructure, resources, and personnel).
3. Identification of cleft care personnel from various specialities whose services can be enrolled in the cleft care network. (Oral surgeons, plastic surgeons,

speech therapists, orthodontists, nutritionists, nurses, paediatricians, ENT specialists, geneticists, psychologists, etc.).

4. Developing a National guideline for timely cleft care (timeline for cleft care, infrastructure, resources, services required for cleft care.)
5. Development of comprehensive software for registry and tracking of patients
6. Capacity building of all statewise service providers
7. Sensitisation of primary healthcare centres (ASHA and Anganwadi workers) on the importance of timely diagnosis, both natal and prenatal, and systematic referral system.
8. Development of decentralised centres for essential services like surgery, orthodontics.
9. Development of centralised centres for online services for rehabilitation like nutrition, speech, and psychology.
10. Development of Govt. funded comprehensive cleft care centres in each state.

Chapter 23
To Sum Up…

Panchali Batra and Sidhi Jain

P. Batra (✉) · S. Jain
Department of Orthodontics, Faculty of Dentistry, Jamia Millia Islamia, New Delhi, India
e-mail: p.batra@jmi.ac.in

P. Batra et al. (eds.), *The Cleft Care Framework in India*,
https://doi.org/10.1007/978-981-99-8968-3_23

S. No.	Name of the Cleft care centres	Year of commencement of Cleft Centre	Cases treated till date	Surgical technique followed	Name of doctor	Contact and email
1.	Sant Parmanand Hospital (New Delhi)	2008	4606	Cleft Lip- Modified Millards repair Cleft Palate- Furlows repair with primary buccal flaps	Dr. Sagar Rajagopal (Centre Head) Dr. Sundereshwer Chander Sood (Plastic Surgeon) Dr. Pankaj Sharma (Oral Surgeon) Dr. Puneet Batra (Orthodontist)	Phone-011-23994401-10 Email-contact@sphdelhi.org
2.	Smile train project, Vivekananda Poly Clinic and Research Institute, (Lucknow, Uttar Pradesh)	2005	9000	Rotation/advancement and its variants (MILLARD), straight line repair (FISCHER), BLACK Procedure, VY procedure, and Bardach's procedure, each with their own specific approaches and modifications for effective correction.	Dr. Amit Agarwal (Centre Head And Plastic Surgeon), Dr. Vaibhav Khanna(Plastic surgeon) Dr.Kamlesh Singh (Orthodontist)	Phone-0522-2321277 Email-deptofplasticsurgeryvpims@gmail.com
3.	Amandeep Hospital, (Amritsar, Punjab)	2010	7680	Cleft Lip- Modified Millard's Technique Cleft Palate- Modified Langenbeck Technique	Dr. Ravi Kumar Mahajan (Plastic Surgeon) Dr. S. S. Kahlon(Orthodontist)	Phone- Mr. Dalbir Singh 9988107272 Mr.Karan: 6280730785 Email-dalbiramandeep@gmail.com

S. No.	Name of the Cleft care centres	Year of commencement of Cleft Centre	Cases treated till date	Surgical technique followed	Name of doctor	Contact and email
4.	Savitri Hospital and Research centre. A Smile Train supported comprehensive cleft care centre. (Gorakhpur, Uttar Pradesh)	1995	>15000	Cleft Lip- Millards Repair Cleft Palate - Furlows and Langenbecks Repair	Dr. Asif Masood (Plastic Surgeon) Dr. Isha Gulati (Orthodontist)	Phone-8604917685 Email-asifmasood64@gmail.com
5.	G S Memorial Plastic Surgery Hospital, (Varanasi, Uttar Pradesh)	2004	40,000	Cleft Lip- Modified Rotation Advancement with small triangular flap and modified triangular flap repair Cleft Palate- Bardach, Furlow's, and Langenbeck	Dr. Subodh Kumar Singh (Centre Head and Plastic Surgeon), Dr. Gaurav Nayyar (plastic Surgeon), Dr. Ishan Singh (Craniomaxillofacial Surgeon) Dr. Abhinav Raj Gupta (Orthodontist)	Phone-8601222230 Email-gsmemorialhospital@gmail.com
6.	CARE CHL Hospital, (Indore, Madhya Pradesh)	2006	9700	Cleft Lip- Modified Millard repair Cleft Palate- Bardach repair	Dr. Jaideep Singh Chauhan (Plastic Surgeon and Project Director) (Dr. Sarwpriya Sharma, (Surgeon) Dr. Virag Bhatia (orthodontist) Dr. Shreyashi Tiwari (Orthodontist)	Phone- +91 9179701455 Email-drjaideepchauhan@gmail.com

S. No.	Name of the Cleft care centres	Year of commencement of Cleft Centre	Cases treated till date	Surgical technique followed	Name of doctor	Contact and email
7.	Sharad Pawar Dental College and Hospital, Acharya Vinobha Bhave Rural Hospital, (Sawangi, Wardha, Maharashtra)	2007		Cleft Lip- Millard rotation advancement flap Cleft Palate- Bardach's Two Flap palatoplasty	Dr. Rajiv Borle(Center Head & Oral and Maxillofacial Surgeon), Dr. Nitin Bhola (Oral and Maxillofacial Surgeon and the Programme Director Smile train), Dr. Ranjit Kamble (Orthodontic treatment coordinator smile train),	Phone-07152 – 287701 Email-ranjitkamble2506@gmail.com
8.	Guwahati Comprehensive Cleft Care Centre (GC4), Mission Smile (Guwahati,Assam)	2011	>20000	For unilateral (Incomplete) cleft lip Fisher's technique, for unilateral (Complete) cleft lip, Modified Mohler's technique and for bilateral (Incomplete & Complete) Millard's technique is used while for incomplete (Unilateral & Bilateral) cleft palate Langenback's technique and for complete (unilateral & Bilateral) palate Bardach's technique is preferred.	Conrad Dennis (Centre Head), Dr. Hiteswar Sarma (Surgeon, Medical Director) Dr Dipjyoti Baruah (Orthodontist).	Phone- +919706091003, +919706091004, +919435016264 Email-contact@missionsmile.org hiteswarsarma@gmail.com
9.	Comprehensive cleft care team at IGIMS, (Patna, Bihar)	2019	500	Millard's rotation advancement flap	Dr. Priyankar Singh (Cleft Surgeon)	Phone-9835378282 Email-spriyankar@yahoo.co.in

S. No.	Name of the Cleft care centres	Year of commencement of Cleft Centre	Cases treated till date	Surgical technique followed	Name of doctor	Contact and email
10.	ABMSS Comprehensive Cleft Care (CCC) Centre, (Kolkata)	2017	1876	Cleft lip- Millard and Fischers technique cleft palate- Bardach's technique and Traditional Vonlagenback's technique for incomplete cleft palate and a Furlows for Submucous cleft palate.	Dr. Siddhartha Chatterjee (Centre's Director) Dr. Rik Mukherjee (Oral and Maxillofacial Surgeon) Dr. Krishnendu Chatterjee (Orthodontist)	Phone- +91 94802 05334 9875448768 Email-info@abmss.in
11.	Ashwini Hospital, (Cuttack, Orissa)	2007	7500	For unilateral cleft lip are Millard's Rotation advancement technique or the Modified Millard's technique, while for bilateral cleft lip Millard's Mulliken technique is used. For primary cleft palate, Von-Langenbeck technique and Bardach's two-flap palatoplasty technique along with Intra Velar Veloplasty are preferred.	Dr. Subrat Kumar Jena (Plastic Surgeon) Dr. Ruchi Gupta (Plastic Surgeon) Dr. Shibani Das (Maxillofacial Surgeon), Dr. Surya Kanta Das (Orthodontist),	Phone-9900460135 Email-smiletrain@ ashwinihospitalcuttack.com
12.	Global Hospital and Research Center, (Mt Abu,Rajasthan)	2001	2500	Cleft lip- Modified Millards repair Cleft palate- Furlows repair with primary buccal flaps	Dr Sharad Mehta (ENT surgeon), DR Keyur Mevada(oral Surgeon) , Dr Puneet Batra (Orthodontist) and Dr Akash Jain (Orthodontist)	Phone-7665408888 Email-info@ghrc-abu.com

S. No.	Name of the Cleft care centres	Year of commencement of Cleft Centre	Cases treated till date	Surgical technique followed	Name of doctor	Contact and email
13.	GSR Institute of Craniofacial and Facial Plastic Surgery (Hyderabad, AndhraPradesh)	1996	35,000	morphofunctional approach for primary lip and palate repair	Dr. Srinivas Gosla Reddy (Plastic Surgeon and Centre Head) Dr. Hemwati Nandan (orthodontist)	Phone- +91 98490 59836 +91 90005 21111 Email-info@ craniofacialinstitute.org
14.	Smile Train, Cleft Leadership Centre, BMJH, (Bangalore, Karnataka)	2005	10,202		Dr. Krishnamurthy Bonanthaya (Oral and Maxillofacial Surgeon & Centre Head), Dr. Dipesh Rao, Dr. Pritham Shetty (Surgeons) Dr. Arvind Sivakumar and Dr. Shruti Bijapur(Orthodontists)	Phone-08041076718 Hotline number- +91 6366-927865 Email-stadminbmj@stclc.com
15.	INGA Health Foundation (Karnataka, West Bengal, Jharkhand, and J&K, Mangalore, Srinagar, and Surat, Bhubaneswar, Mumbai, Vizag, Patna, and Agra).	2006	9974	cleft lip- Modified Millards Rotation Advancement Cheiloplasty cleft palate- Bardach and Salyer Technique, and Von-Langenbeck technique	Dr. Krishna Shama Rao and Dr. Chetana Kumar (craniofacial Surgeons and Centre Heads) Dr. Rolson Sandeep Amanna, Dr. Tarun Jain, Dr. Lohitha Kurupati Krishna (Craniofacial Surgeons) Dr. Aparajita (an Orthodontist)	Phone-9741983160 Email-drchetana@ingahealth. org

S. No.	Name of the Cleft care centres	Year of commencement of Cleft Centre	Cases treated till date	Surgical technique followed	Name of doctor	Contact and email
16.	Centre For Craniofacial Anomalies, (Mangalore, Karnataka)	2010	1708	Afzore technique for cleft lip and palate correction	Dr. Akhter Husain(Cleft Orthodontist & Director) Dr. H. Hari Kishore Bhat (Oral and Maxillofacial Surgeon & Project Director) Dr. Srinivas Gosla Reddy (Visiting Craniofacial Consultant)	Phone-0824-2206000 ext 2268, 2272 9632959390 8496962992 Email-craniofacial@ yenepoya.edu.in
17.	The Cleft and Craniofacial Centre, Sree Balaji Medical College & Hospital and Dr Rela Institute (Chennai, Tamil Nadu)	2022			Dr. Syed Altaf Hussain (Plastic Surgeon & Centre Head), Dr Charanya Vijayakumar (Oral and Maxillofacial Surgeon), Dr Badri Thiruvenkatachari (Orthodontist), Dr Manoj Pratap C (Orthodontist), Dr Subhiksha (Orthodontist)	Phone-044 6666 7806 9566230075 +91 446666 7806 (Landline) +919566230075 + 91 96 0006 3199 (Mobile) Email- cleftcraniofacialcentre@ gmail.com cleftcraniofacial@outlook.in, sa_hussain@hotmail.com

S. No.	Name of the Cleft care centres	Year of commencement of Cleft Centre	Cases treated till date	Surgical technique followed	Name of doctor	Contact and email
18.	ABMSS Comprehensive Cleft Care (CCC) Centre, (Bangalore, Karnataka)	2018	1157	Cleft lip- Fischers anatomic subunit technique Bardach's 2 flap with Buccal fat pad for the raw area coverage in complete cleft palate, wardill kilner technique or Traditional Vonlagenback's technique for incomplete cleft palate and Furlows for Submucous cleft palate.	Dr. Jayanth B S(Oral and Maxillofacial Surgeon & Centre Head), Dr. Shobha Hegde (Maxillofacial Surgeon), Dr. Gautam (orthodontist), Dr. Prajwal (Orthodontist),	Phone- +91 94802 05334 8048148651 Email-info@abmss.in
19.	ABMSS Comprehensive Cleft Care (CCC) Centre, (Hyderabad, AndhraPradesh)	2015	2000	Cleft lip- Modified Millard and Afroz'e Technique Veau-Wardill-Kilner, Von Langenback's V-Y Pushback technique for incomplete cleft palate and a Furlows for Submucous cleft palate.	Dr. Dushyant Prasad (Founder), Dr. Vijay Kumar (Maxillofacial Surgeon) Dr. Nikita Reddy (Orthodontist)	Phone- +91 94802 05334 Email-info@abmss.in

MIX
Papier aus verantwortungsvollen Quellen
Paper from responsible sources
FSC® C105338
FSC
www.fsc.org

If you have any concerns about our products,
you can contact us on
ProductSafety@springernature.com

In case Publisher is established outside the EU,
the EU authorized representative is:
Springer Nature Customer Service Center GmbH
Europaplatz 3, 69115 Heidelberg, Germany

Printed by Libri Plureos GmbH
in Hamburg, Germany